PCOS Diet

---

*The Complete Guide to Fight PCOS,
Prevent Diabetes, Lose Weight and
Increase Fertility*

By Brad Clark

from various sources. Please consult a licensed professional before attempting any techniques outlined in this book.

By reading this document, the reader agrees that under no circumstances is the author responsible for any losses, direct or indirect, that are incurred as a result of the use of information contained within this document, including, but not limited to, errors, omissions, or inaccuracies.

Introduction: Polycystic Ovary Syndrome

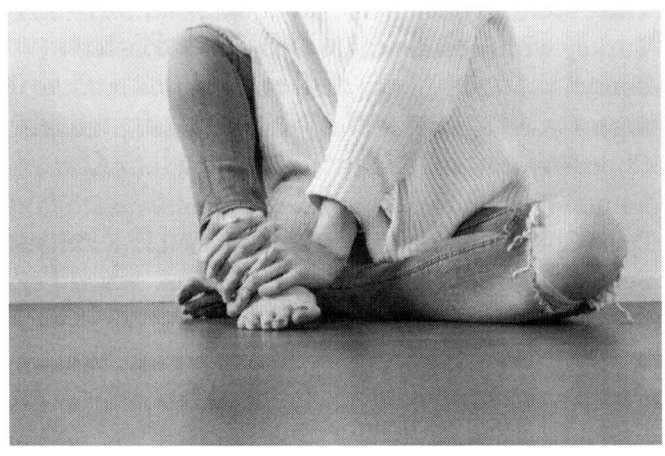

Polycystic Ovarian Syndrome or PCOS is a type of hormonal disorder that commonly occurs in women of reproductive age. When you suffer from this condition, you may experience prolonged or infrequent menstrual periods. In some cases, you could have excessively high levels of androgens—hormones typically associated with the male reproductive system.

Women with PCOS may develop collections of follicles (fluid) and aren't able to release eggs regularly. Many women suffer from this condition without even knowing it. PCOS mainly affects the ovaries—the reproductive organs responsible for producing progesterone and estrogen. These are the hormones in charge of the menstrual cycle's regulation. Normally, the ovaries also produce small amounts of androgens.

Women's ovaries release eggs regularly for fertilization. An egg is released each month through a process known as ovulation. The hormones in charge of ovulation are the luteinizing hormone (LH) and the follicle-stimulating hormone (FSH). The FSH hormone is in charge of stimulating the ovary so it produces a follicle—an egg-containing sac—while the LH stimulates the ovary so that it releases a mature egg.

PCOS is considered a syndrome—a collection of symptoms affecting ovulation and the ovaries. The main characteristics of PCOS are:

- Cyst formation in the ovaries

- Skipped or irregular periods

- Abnormally high levels of androgens

When you suffer from this condition, several small sacs filled with fluid grow within your ovaries. In fact, the term "polycystic" literally means "many cysts." Actually, these sacs are follicles that contain immature eggs. These eggs don't reach maturity to stimulate ovulation. When this happens, your hormone levels are altered, giving you abnormally low levels of female hormones and abnormally high levels of male hormones. This, in turn, disrupts your menstrual cycle, which is why you could experience fewer menstrual periods than usual. Here are the other effects PCOS may have on your body:

- Depression

When you experience all the hormonal symptoms and bodily changes of PCOS, this can have an adverse effect on your emotions. A lot of women who have PCOS also end up experiencing anxiety and depression because of their condition.

- Endometrial Cancer

Normally, when you menstruate, you also shed your uterine lining. However, if you don't menstruate regularly, this may cause an accumulation of your uterine lining, which increases your risk of developing endometrial cancer.

- Infertility

You can't get pregnant if you don't ovulate. When you don't experience regular ovulation, your ovaries aren't releasing eggs for sperm to fertilize. This is why PCOS is one of the main causes of infertility.

- Metabolic Syndrome (MS)

Most women who suffer from PCOS are either obese or overweight. This is a huge problem, because both PCOS and obesity increase your risk for low HDL levels and high levels of LDL cholesterol, blood pressure, and blood sugar. When you experience all of these, you find yourself at risk for metabolic syndrome—which, in turn, increases your risk of stroke, heart disease, and diabetes.

- Sleep Apnea

PCOS sufferers may experience frequent pauses in their breathing while sleeping. This condition, which often interrupts restful sleep, is known as sleep apnea—and it's more common in women who have PCOS and are overweight.

What Causes PCOS?

Right now, nobody knows the exact cause of the condition known as PCOS. But there are certain risk factors that may increase your likelihood of developing this condition. These risk factors include:

- Genetics

If you have any relatives—especially a sister or a mother—with PCOS, there is a higher likelihood that you would develop this condition, as well. Genetics is one of the main risk factors of this difficult condition.

- Excessive amounts of insulin

Insulin is one of the body's hormones produced by the pancreas. It allows the cells to utilize sugar—the main energy supply of the body. When your cells develop a resistance to insulin, your levels of blood sugar might increase which, in turn, causes your body to produce more insulin. When you have excessive levels of insulin, this increases the production of androgen, thus causing issues with your ovulation.

- Excessively High Levels of Androgen

This happens when the ovaries start producing more androgens than normal, and may result in acne and hirsutism.

- Inflammation (Low-Grade)

This refers to when white blood cells start producing substances in an attempt to combat infection. According to research, PCOS sufferers have a specific kind of low-grade inflammation that triggers the ovaries to start producing androgens, leading to problems with the blood vessels and the heart.

When you suffer from PCOS, this places you at risk for a number of other health concerns such as:

- Abnormal bleeding of the uterus
- Anxiety
- Endometrial cancer
- Gestational diabetes
- Heart attacks
- High blood pressure
- High cholesterol

- Increased amount of lipids

- Infertility

- Liver disease

- Metabolic syndrome

- Miscarriage

- Obesity that may lead to low self-esteem or depression

- Sleep apnea

- Steatohepatitis or nonalcoholic fatty liver

- Type 2 diabetes

The Symptoms of PCOS

The symptoms of PCOS may start developing during puberty—right around the time when you get your first period. However, there are times when PCOS may develop later in life, for instance, because you have gained a substantial amount of weight. While the symptoms of this condition may vary from one person to another, in order for a doctor to diagnose PCOS, you must manifest at least two of the following:

- Acne

Excessive amounts of male hormones make the skin oilier which, in turn, causes breakouts of the face, upper back, and chest.

- Excess androgen

When you have excessive levels of androgens, this may manifest in the form of excess body and facial hair, severe acne, and even male-pattern baldness in some cases.

- Headaches

Hormonal changes may trigger frequent headaches in some PCOS sufferers.

- Irregular menstrual periods

Prolonged, infrequent, or irregular menstrual cycles are very common in women suffering from PCOS. For instance, you may have less than nine menstrual periods each year, more than 35 days between your menstrual periods, or when you do have your period, it's always abnormally heavy.

When you don't experience regular ovulation, this prevents you from regularly shedding your uterine lining. Then, when your uterine lining accumulates for a long period of time, your periods become heavier than usual.

- Polycystic ovaries

Those who suffer from PCOS may have enlarged ovaries that contain follicles surrounding the eggs. This results in a failure to function properly.

- Skin darkening

Sometimes, you may start noticing your skin becoming darker, especially in the creases of your body like those in the groin, neck, and under your breasts.

- Weight gain

Approximately 80% of women who suffer from PCOS are either obese or overweight.

Knowing the symptoms of PCOS makes you more aware of the condition. And once you notice these symptoms, you can have yourself checked to see whether or not you suffer from PCOS. Such helpful information can enrich your life—and you can also help enrich the lives of others by leaving a positive review for this book to guide them to the same information! Of course, there is still more to learn. Read on!

Chapter 1: The PCOS Diet

PCOS is a common irreversible condition that comes with permanent effects like diabetes and infertility when left untreated or unmanaged. But with the proper lifestyle and diet, you have the potential to put your condition into remission. Following a healthy diet and lifestyle can even help bring balance to your hormones so that you can conceive naturally. While there are different types of PCOS, the most recognized ones are:

- Insulin-Resistant

This is the most common type of PCOS, characterized by high levels of insulin that impede ovulation. Excessively high levels of insulin delay ovulation while promoting an increase in testosterone levels. When you have reached child-bearing years and you don't ovulate regularly, your body won't be able to make sufficient amounts of progesterone and estradiol to balance your testosterone out.

When you have become insulin-resistant, your body becomes less sensitive to insulin surges that are released after you eat. This, in turn, causes your body to produce more and more insulin until your muscles and liver respond. Insulin-resistant PCOS is commonly caused by a poor diet, environmental toxins, and stress.

- Inflammation-Based

This type of PCOS results from chronic inflammation of the body's systems. This is more difficult to manage than insulin-resistant PCOS because sufferers typically experience other health issues like joint pain, intestinal permeability or a leaky gut, skin conditions, and other types of inflammation biomarkers. When you experience chronic inflammation, your ovulation may stop, as well. Inflammation-based PCOS is typically caused by an inflammatory diet, stress, and environmental toxins.

- Synthetic Hormone-Induced

This type of PCOS is sometimes called "post-pill PCOS," as it occurs when women go off their hormonal birth control pills. Since you aren't producing hormones while on these pills because the pills supply the artificial hormones for you, when you stop taking them, your body loses its natural ability for hormone production. This happens when your ovaries lose contact with your pituitary gland. When you no longer have artificial hormones and your body isn't able to produce these hormones naturally, you may develop this condition.

One of the most effective ways to prevent or manage PCOS—or even put it into remission—is by following a specific diet known as the PCOS diet. Basically, while on this diet, you would have to:

- Limit your intake of dairy

- Avoid eating gluten

- Increase your intake of lean protein

- Reduce your sugar intake

- Consume enough amounts of fiber

- Consume a lot of whole foods

Apart from these basic food rules, there are other things you must keep in mind while following the PCOS diet. We will be going through these rules, tips, and strategies throughout the chapters of this book. That way, you will be able to understand them more within the context of the topics covered. For now, keep these simple rules in mind as part of your new PCOS diet:

- Breakfast is the most important meal of the day—so you shouldn't miss it

If you are used to skipping breakfast, you should stop this habit right now because it is aggravating your condition. While it's okay to skip breakfast once in a while, you should make it a point to consume a healthy meal within one hour after you wake up in the morning.

- Spice up your life!

Adding spices into your meals or recipes can enhance their detoxification effects. Most spices help promote natural detoxification processes, so don't be afraid to add these in when cooking.

- Eliminate anything that has adverse effects on your hormones or hormone levels

These include alcohol, caffeine, and refined sugar. All foods and beverages containing these three things tend to deplete the essential nutrients in your body—especially those which support your fertility. It's also recommended to reduce your dairy intake as much as possible.

- Focus on foods that are low on the glycemic index

To do this, you may have to incorporate more plant-based whole foods such as veggies, fruits, whole grains, legumes, and nuts. You should also opt for healthy sources of fat instead of refined fats. Lean protein is important, too, so make sure that you focus on such foods. While following the

PCOS diet, you should avoid processed foods, refined flours, and sugar.

- Eat healthy foods that will make your cells happy

While the liver is the main organ that detoxifies the body, you should make sure that your gut is healthy, too. There are specific nutrients these detoxifying organs and systems required to function well. While following the PCOS diet, you should get yourself checked regularly to make sure you are eating a balanced diet and aren't developing any nutrient deficiencies.

- Take supplements—as needed

Speaking of deficiencies, you might not be able to get all the nutrients your body needs from the food you eat. While it's better to acquire all these nutrients from food, if you can't, then you might have to start taking supplements. Some examples of supplements suggested for those suffering from PCOS are:

- **CoQ10** improves ovulation and reproductive function.

- **Maca** helps support the balance of hormones.

○ **Magnesium** supports the detoxification of the liver and promotes insulin activity.

○ **Myoinositol** helps lower levels of testosterone, restore menstrual cycles, and improve the functions of the ovaries.

○ **NAC** helps improve insulin sensitivity and detoxification processes.

○ **Vitamin B12** helps promote the detoxification of the liver.

○ **Vitamin D** helps support the development of eggs and insulin action.

The Pros and Cons of the PCOS Diet

Apart from following the PCOS diet, making healthier lifestyle choices can also help improve your condition. Sadly, when you are diagnosed with PCOS, doctors usually first suggest that you take medications. While you might experience improvements after taking medication, following a healthier diet and lifestyle is much more effective and better for your overall well-being. With these healthy changes, you won't have to take medications which may have potential side effects.

One of the primary biochemical issues behind this condition is insulin resistance. For women who suffer from PCOS, their bodies think there is a deficiency of insulin thus, they produce more. When this happens, it sets off a chain reaction, and one of the effects is an increase in the production of male hormones. Most women who suffer from PCOS are also overweight or obese— and this is linked to insulin resistance, as well. Therefore, women with PCOS find that gaining weight is much easier than shedding excess pounds.

When you suffer from this condition, don't just focus on losing weight—you must also learn how to manage your insulin resistance. As a condition, insulin resistance makes you gain weight faster whether you also have PCOS or not. When you learn how to manage this condition, weight loss may soon follow. And some research has shown that losing a reasonable amount of weight may improve your response to certain fertility treatments. So where does the PCOS diet come in?

Most evidence shows that the PCOS diet—which recommends consuming moderate amounts of carbs—may help you manage your condition. During your meal planning, make sure you include non-starchy veggies, healthy protein, and other types of nutrient-rich foods. When making changes to your diet, it's important for you to find your "sweet spot" where you feel happy and satisfied. That way, you won't abandon your new diet after a short time because you feel it's too difficult.

Probably one of the most significant downsides of the PCOS diet is that most women aren't able to find this sweet spot. Since the diet does have some specific rules and recommendations, some women tend to focus too much on what they shouldn't eat and, after some time, they start feeling bad about themselves.

One of the main issues is limiting carbs. For most people, carbs are the main source of fuel. However, most of us consume more than our bodies need. Of course, any excess that isn't used by the body gets stored as fat. And the more we eat, the more weight we gain. This is why it's extremely important for you to find your own healthy balance that you can sustain in the long run.

One of the great benefits of the PCOS diet is that it's not a one-size-fits-all kind of diet. As long as you know the rules, recommendations, and guidelines, you can develop your own PCOS diet that you feel comfortable with. You can also work together with your doctor or nutritionist to design your diet so you can get input from other sources.

When it comes to the PCOS diet, there is no set time-frame as to when you will start experiencing improvements in your condition. This varies from one person to another. A lot of women may experience weight loss, an improvement in the health of their skin, and a more regular period within one month after starting the PCOS diet. And the longer you stick with it, the more improvements you will see!

The Benefits of the PCOS Diet

The sad thing about PCOS is that it doesn't go away. But even if there isn't any cure for PCOS—at least in terms of medication—following the PCOS diet can help prevent complications and reduce the symptoms. This is great news for all PCOS sufferers because compared to other popular diets, the PCOS diet is quite flexible. When implementing the PCOS diet, focus on making a few small changes at a time. This makes it easier for your body to adjust to the diet and it also allows you to "wean" yourself off any unhealthy foods you love—but that aren't recommended for the diet. If you're still on the fence about the PCOS diet, here are some benefits you may look forward to:

1. Weight loss

Reducing the amount of carbs you eat per day helps promote weight loss—especially if you're used to following a high-carb diet. More and more studies have confirmed that the main benefit of moderate- or low-carb diet is weight loss. More than other types of foods, carbs trigger the release of insulin—the main hormone of the body that stores fat. And since PCOS already increases your insulin production, reducing your carb intake becomes even more important. Also, weight loss is the first benefit you will start experiencing after a month or so of following the PCOS diet.

2. Improvement of hormone-related problems

PCOS is mainly associated with the disruption of hormonal balance, and most of the symptoms of this condition occur because of this imbalance. Hormonal imbalances are influenced by how much insulin your body produces and how much you actually weigh. Sadly, this is only one aspect of the condition, as it also disrupts the regulation and production of insulin along with the metabolic functions linked to the maintenance of a healthy weight.

Most people who suffer from PCOS have issues with insulin regulation which, if left unchecked, might lead to prediabetes or even type 2 diabetes once they reach middle age. This, and other hormonal imbalances, may increase your risk of high blood pressure, heart disease, and some types of cancers.

But when you eat foods low on the glycemic index and reduce your carb intake, this can help bring balance to your hormones. Depending on other issues you are experiencing, you may want to adjust your protein and fat intake, as well. This is why you may want to start counting calories, especially at the beginning of your PCOS diet journey. Over time, you will be able to determine if what you have eaten—and how much you have eaten—is enough for the day. Studies have shown that weight loss—the first benefit of the PCOS diet—can improve your symptoms while reducing your risk of other health issues.

3. Reduce inflammation

PCOS and obesity are associated with inflammation. PCOS sufferers are more likely to be obese, which is associated with inflammation, and inflammation may worsen—and even cause— PCOS. It's a vicious cycle that you can break with a healthy diet. According to research, the PCOS diet can reduce inflammation, help you lose weight, and help you maintain a healthy weight. It's also helpful for managing the various symptoms of the condition. In particular, this benefit can also support your reproductive health.

4. Calm down your stomach

When you significantly reduce your carb intake, you may experience fewer stomach issues. Usually, there will be less risk of stomach cramps, diarrhea, and gas. In a lot of cases, women also experience less heartburn.

5. Reduce acne

A lot of women also experience improvement in the health of their skin while following the PCOS diet. Modern research has shown there is a direct connection between acne and high-carb diets, due to the effect of carb-rich foods on IGF, insulin, and other growth hormones. If you want to improve your acne and other skin conditions, you may want to start lowering your carb intake—and your dairy intake, as well.

Aside from offering physical benefits to PCOS sufferers, research has shown that following the PCOS diet may also provide positive psychological effects. The more you start noticing the benefits of this diet, the happier and more satisfied you will feel. And since the PCOS diet can be customized according to your own needs and preferences, you won't have to feel too stressed about following it!

How Does the PCOS Diet Differ From Other Diets?

When followed correctly, lifestyle and diet changes are a lot more effective than PCOS medications. In fact, one particular study showed that the pregnancy rates for common PCOS medications were less than 15%, while the rate for lifestyle changes and the PCOS diet was a whopping 20%! This is a huge deal and it's extremely exciting news for a lot of PCOS sufferers, because infertility is one of the most devastating symptoms of this condition.

Why is this relevant?

Higher pregnancy rates show that these women have ovulated. This, in turn, means that they have—through a healthier lifestyle and the PCOS diet—successfully balanced their hormones. Their testosterone levels have decreased and they were able to control their insulin levels, as well. So, if you continue these healthy habits long-term, you can expect weight loss, acne improvements, and a decrease in excess hair growth—and other benefits are soon to come, as well.

When you first learn about the different rules and guidelines of the PCOS diet, you might think of it as restrictive. But the more you customize the diet and the more you start feeling its great benefits, you will come to realize that starting the PCOS diet is the best thing you could have done for your condition. While it may take some extra time and effort to prepare your own meals each day to ensure that you are only eating healthy dishes appropriate for your diet, over time, things will become easier—and you will be able to do meal prepping a lot faster.

A lot of other diets and diet trends these days claim that they are the healthiest ones and can help you manage different conditions. While this may be true for other types of conditions, when you suffer from PCOS, a personalized and recommended eating plan—the PCOS diet—will be much more beneficial for you. What makes the PCOS diet different from other diets is that it's a combination of the following:

- Anti-inflammatory diets

- High-fat, low-carb diets (like the ketogenic diet)

- Low-calorie, weight loss diets

- Low-glycemic index diets

Aside from managing the symptoms of PCOS, the PCOS diet also helps improve other conditions because of all the benefits it offers. By working with a nutritionist or doctor to come up with your own PCOS diet plan specifically tailored to your preferences and needs, you will be able to get the most out of this diet. This is a person-centered approach to dieting, which makes this diet much more appealing than other eating plans.

Chapter 2: The PCOS Diet and Other Conditions

Learning how to manage PCOS can feel quite overwhelming and frustrating at times. This hormonal condition can cause you to experience some adverse symptoms that might make you feel like you've lost control of your own body. If you suffer from PCOS, you may have already done a lot of research about it—and about how you can manage it more effectively. We have already established that the PCOS diet can help you with this condition, but a healthy diet can also reduce your insulin resistance and help improve other issues, as well.

Following the PCOS diet entails finding the right balance of foods that contain healthy nutrients. It includes a wide range of fruits, vegetables, legumes, whole grains, lean proteins, healthy fats, and minimal amounts of carbs and dairy products. It's also recommended to avoid excessive amounts of sodium, saturated fats, trans fats, and sugars in all forms.

A balanced and healthy diet is recommended when you suffer from PCOS, because such a diet allows you to incorporate foods that are low on the glycemic index. Such foods take a longer time to digest, which means they raise your levels of blood sugar gradually instead of causing them to spike. Conversely, when you eat a lot of foods high on the glycemic index, this causes your body to produce more insulin, thus aggravating your condition.

While you will have to limit your intake of certain foods, you don't have to eliminate entire food groups when on the PCOS diet. This is one thing PCOS sufferers love about the diet. It's not really restrictive, it just helps you learn how to have a healthier relationship with food. Now, let's take a look at how PCOS and other health conditions are connected—and how the diet can help.

The PCOS Diet and Diabetes

Some studies have suggested that when you suffer from insulin resistance, this creates an adverse reaction that involves your endocrine system. Over time, this may lead to the development of type 2 diabetes. This type of diabetes is characterized by the body's cells being resistant to insulin or the body's excessive production of insulin. Right now, more than 30 million people in America suffer from this condition and from other forms of diabetes, too.

It's important to note that both conditions have their own specific treatments, which may either offset or complement one another. Let's say, for instance, you have PCOS and you are taking birth control pills. In some cases, these pills may help clear up your acne and regulate your menstrual periods. But there are some types of birth control pills that increase your blood sugar levels—which is definitely an issue if you're at risk for developing diabetes. There are also certain medications for type 2 diabetes that may help improve insulin resistance—which is beneficial for when you suffer from PCOS.

Typically, type 2 diabetes is manageable or preventable through a proper diet and physical exercise. Research has shown that PCOS is one of the risk factors for the development of diabetes. As a matter of fact, women who get PCOS even before their child-bearing years have a higher risk of developing diabetes later in life. PCOS sufferers are up to eight times more likely to develop this condition than non-PCOS sufferers. Obesity is another significant risk factor—which also happens to be one of the effects of PCOS.

Since the PCOS diet can help you manage the condition more effectively, it may also help you manage—or even prevent—diabetes. Pairing this incredible diet with regular exercise is even more beneficial, because physical activity helps you burn excess blood sugar while promoting the cells' insulin sensitivity. When this happens, your body becomes more effective at utilizing insulin. Therefore, the PCOS diet and exercise benefits both conditions—while allowing you to maintain a healthy weight, too. Here are some tips for following the PCOS diet to improve PCOS and diabetes:

- Eat foods that have anti-inflammatory effects

Both conditions are associated with chronic inflammation. Therefore, consuming a lot of anti-inflammatory foods may help reduce inflammation in your body while improving insulin resistance, as well. Some studies have shown that anti-inflammatory diets may lead to weight loss, as well as a reduction in PCOS symptoms.

- Eat a lot of foods that promote weight loss

There are many foods that promote weight loss and are suitable for the PCOS diet. If you want to manage PCOS and diabetes better, losing weight—even a little bit at a time—will go a long way. Apart from making healthier food choices, try reducing your portion intake at each meal, too. Over time, these small changes will make a difference.

- Choose spices and flavor enhancers wisely

There are certain spices that may help improve insulin sensitivity, lower blood sugar levels, fight inflammation, and reduce PCOS or diabetes symptoms. Some of these spices include cinnamon, turmeric, black pepper, ginger, fennel, chili peppers, and more.

- If you have to eat carbs, opt for healthy carb sources

While you should lower your overall carb intake, you don't have to eliminate carbs from your diet altogether. Make sure you go for healthy sources such as whole grains, raw veggies, fresh fruits, and dairy products with reduced fat.

- Avoid processed and junk foods

In order to get the most out of the PCOS diet, one of the best things to do is avoid any processed, packaged, or junk food. Remember that you have decided to follow this diet in order to live a healthier life. Cutting out these types of food items will help you reach your health goals faster.

PCOS and the risk of developing diabetes go together, but you don't have to surrender to either one. You can combat these conditions with these diet strategies and healthier lifestyle choices. When it comes to making positive changes to your life, start with small adjustments and follow your instincts. Soon, you will see—and feel—the improvements happening in your life.

The PCOS Diet and Weight Loss

When you find out that you have PCOS—whether you have mild or severe symptoms—thinking about what you should do next can be a challenge. Although this condition is linked to insulin production and hormone levels, don't blame yourself for developing the condition. Difficult as it may be, try to look on the bright side of things and remember that you can manage—and even improve—the condition with the help of the PCOS diet.

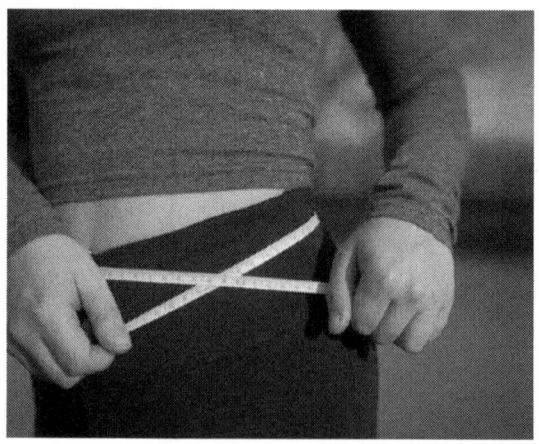

When it comes to the PCOS diet and weight loss, there's more to it than just eating less to shed excess pounds. When you suffer from PCOS, your body has developed insulin resistance. This leads to weight gain, and when you have excess body fat, this increases your body's insulin production—which, in turn, aggravates your condition. This creates a vicious cycle that makes it seem virtually impossible to lose weight.

However, it only *seems* impossible. With the right knowledge and strategies, you can start losing those stubborn pounds little by little in order to improve your conditions. Here are some weight-loss tips for you when following the PCOS diet:

- Focus more on health, not just on the food you eat

Instead of focusing on "dieting," you should think about "being healthy." This gives you the proper mindset to make the PCOS diet more sustainable for you. Try consuming a lot of whole foods, veggies, fruits, and other low-GI foods to prevent spikes in your blood sugar levels. You can think of PCOS as your body's way of telling you you can't handle high levels of sugar. Making changes in your diet is an effective way to change your life for the better—and it can help you become healthier in the future, too.

- Don't be afraid of fats or carbs

Many PCOS sufferers are scared of fats and carbs because they don't want to gain more weight.

However, as long as you choose healthy fat and carb sources that will keep you full and satisfied, you won't have to worry about including these macros in your diet. Eliminating certain food groups from your diet might throw your body off balance and worsen your condition. That's why it's recommended to make small changes so your body adjusts more easily.

- Try to balance your blood sugar levels throughout the day

This is an important tip that you should consciously incorporate into your daily life. Start with a healthy breakfast filled with low-GI foods that your body will break down slowly—until your next meal. Make sure to choose meals that will stabilize your blood sugar levels. Such meals include healthy fats, proteins, and healthy carbs.

- Be aware of foods that disrupt your hormones

When your body is already struggling to bring balance to your hormonal levels, the last thing you want to consume are foods that cause further disruption to these hormones. Additionally, you should avoid other factors that may disrupt your hormonal balance such as not getting enough sleep, not knowing how to manage stress, using BPA-containing plastic containers, and more.

The PCOS Diet and Infertility

Another common effect of PCOS that can be devastating to those who suffer from it is infertility. Some experience difficulty conceiving while others aren't able to conceive at all, depending on the severity of the condition. PCOS is one of the main causes of infertility, and this happens because women have irregular ovulation and menstrual periods. The hormonal imbalances prevent mature eggs from developing and being released, which means ovulation and pregnancy cannot occur. Even if women ovulate, this hormonal imbalance prevents the mature eggs from being properly implanted.

Although PCOS doesn't have a cure, it is a manageable condition—and one way to cope with it is through the PCOS diet. While there are different kinds of medications that may help with infertility, focusing on weight loss and proper nutrition can improve PCOS outcomes. In fact, a 10% weight reduction may already promote your regular menstrual cycle—and when you start having periods regularly, this improves your chances of getting pregnant. Also, following the PCOS diet, which is low in sugar, doesn't just help you lose weight, but it also slows down the progression of the condition in order to prevent the development of type 2 diabetes.

Even though changing your diet can be a challenge—especially if this is your first time following any kind of healthy diet—think about the perks! If you suffer from PCOS and your doctor has informed you that you're having difficulties conceiving because of this condition, know that this diet can help you turn things around. Making small yet meaningful changes in your diet—gradually shifting to the PCOS diet—allows you to improve your health and increase your chances of getting pregnant.

Chapter 3: Starting Your PCOS Diet Journey

By now, you already know that the PCOS diet can help improve your condition. Whether you have just discovered that you suffer from this condition or you have already known for some time, starting the diet is key to start controlling it. While the exact cause of PCOS isn't known, the best thing you can do is manage your symptoms through the healthy PCOS diet.

Starting your PCOS diet journey involves knowing the kinds of foods recommended for you to eat. That way, you can plan your meals around these foods, making it much easier for you to follow. To help you out, here is some basic information about the recommended foods for this special diet—along with a few general pointers, too:

- Eat small, frequent meals

This may help promote healthy energy and blood sugar levels as well as weight loss. When planning your small meals, make sure to include healthy foods such as:

○ Fiber

This helps slow down digestion to prevent blood sugar spikes. Fiber also promotes satiety, which is key for controlling caloric intake and reducing appetite. You can get fiber from whole grains, beans, leafy green vegetables, and more.

○ Healthy fats

These are essential for your overall health. Healthy fats have anti-inflammatory properties, balance blood sugar, and promote satiety. You can get healthy fats from nuts, avocados, and plant-based oils.

○ Protein

This is an essential nutrient for promoting weight management, satiety, and balanced levels of blood sugar. There are plenty of healthy plant-based protein sources such as beans, nut butters, nuts, edamame, tofu, and more. You can also consume lean meats to get enough protein.

- Drink fresh juices and smoothies

An easy, effective, and low-calorie way to consume more nutrients is by drinking fresh juice and smoothies. Although processed juices may contain high amounts of sugar, you can make your own fresh juice from real fruits and veggies.

That way, you don't have to worry about added sugars since you are choosing the ingredients for your homemade juice and smoothie drinks.

- Reduce your caffeine intake

This might come as a surprise to a lot of people, because caffeinated drinks—like coffee and tea—have some significant health benefits. However, caffeine tends to reduce your insulin sensitivity, which isn't ideal when you suffer from PCOS. Rather than drinking caffeinated beverages, you may opt for water infused with ginger or lemon, caffeine-free tea and coffee beverages, and more.

- Get your levels of vitamin D checked regularly

This tip is important because you shouldn't allow yourself to develop a deficiency in vitamin D. A deficiency in this particular vitamin is linked to insulin resistance, therefore, you must avoid it. Having yourself checked regularly allows you to determine if you need to start taking vitamin D supplements.

When it comes to the PCOS diet, you should be reasonably strict with yourself. This is one of the hardest things you may have to do—especially at the beginning. But the more you stick with it, the more you will start experiencing the wonderful effects of this diet. And the more you learn about this diet, the more you understand how to follow it properly. If you find the information in this book helpful and enlightening, you may want to leave a positive review for others to start their PCOS diet journey, as well. This is one journey all PCOS sufferers must take, as it will improve your life in the long run.

How to Start the PCOS Diet

The basic rule and guideline for following the PCOS diet is to focus on whole foods, plant-based food sources, and fresh proteins while limiting your intake of trans fats, sugars, and processed foods. Depending on your own health goals and needs, you may have to calculate your macros or even take supplements as recommended by your doctor. If you're wondering how to start the PCOS diet, here is a general list of guidelines. Use this as a starting point, but you may also think of your own rules or consult with professionals to help you out:

- First, know your reason for starting the diet

If you want to increase your success on the PCOS diet, you should know why you want to start it in the first place. Of course, you want to improve your PCOS symptoms, but if you have other reasons beyond that—like wanting to adopt a healthier lifestyle—this will make you more motivated to stick with the change. If you think it will help, make a list of all your reasons for following the PCOS diet. And every time you feel like giving up, go back to that list to find your motivation once again.

- Clean up your environment and stock up on healthy foods

Another way to increase your chances of sticking with the PCOS diet is by removing any temptations from your environment—meaning, your home. Start by cleaning up your kitchen. Go through all of your cupboards and get rid of foods that aren't beneficial to your condition such as white rice, pasta, potatoes, chips, biscuits, chocolates, processed foods, processed meat, and sugary beverages. You don't have to throw these foods out—just donate them! After you have cleaned up your kitchen and pantry, stock up on healthy, PCOS-friendly foods like:

- Fresh produce like non-starchy fruits and veggies.

- Full-fat dairy products which you can enjoy occasionally.

- Whole grains.

- Avoid skipping meals

Remember the tip about eating small, frequent meals? When you have set regular mealtimes for yourself, try to avoid skipping meals as much as possible. That way, your blood sugar levels don't go down to dangerous levels. Also, it's recommended to have at least two to three hours between your meals to allow your body to process the food you have eaten.

When starting the PCOS diet, finding support can also help you out in a big way. When you are able to talk with other people who suffer from the same condition and who started the PCOS diet before you, it's easier for you to make the transition. You can also get real-life tips from other women who have found success in the PCOS diet and who have come up with their own effective tips that you may employ, as well.

PCOS Diet Shopping List

Meal planning is an important part of the PCOS diet—and any other kind of special diet, as well. Planning your meals allows you to guide yourself throughout each week so you can make sure you're getting all the nutrients your body needs each day. This also helps you ensure you don't eat too little—or too much. When you suffer from PCOS, following the PCOS diet is an excellent way to take control of your condition instead of allowing it to take control of you. Here is a sample PCOS diet shopping list for you—along with some tips on where you can find these food items and how you can use them in your recipes:

- Anti-inflammatory ingredients

When cooking or prepping meals for your PCOS diet, make sure to include a lot of anti-inflammatory ingredients. These ingredients make your meals healthier as they reduce inflammation in your body. Some examples of anti-inflammatory ingredients are:

○ Apple cider vinegar

○ Matcha powder

○ MCT oil

○ Herbs and spices like cinnamon, turmeric, parsley, and more

These are common ingredients that add flavor to your recipes along with a healthy boost of nutrients. You can get these from different retailers, both online and in physical stores.

- Fresh produce

When choosing food items and ingredients for your PCOS diet, you can't go wrong with fresh produce—especially the non-starchy varieties. Fresh fruits and veggies contain a wide range of nutrients along with some excellent health benefits. Some examples of fresh produce for your diet include:

○ Apples

○ Kiwis

○ Berries (strawberries, blueberries, blackberries, raspberries)

○ Lemons

○ Pineapples

○ Tomatoes

○ Broccoli

- Cauliflower

- Dark, leafy veggies like spinach and kale

- Grains

Instead of consuming refined carbs like pasta, bread, and white rice, you can opt for whole grains that are high in fiber. If you're a carb-lover, choosing healthier carb sources can make your PCOS diet journey a lot easier. Opt for mineral-rich grains that your body digests at a slower rate. This allows you to continue eating the carbs you love while still staying healthy and fit. Some examples of these healthy grains you can purchase from grocery and health food stores are:

- Quinoa

- Brown rice

- Whole-wheat bread

- Sorghum (if your local shops don't have this, you can buy it online, too)

- Healthy fats

Essential fatty acids are considered "essential" because they help improve our body's ability to absorb other nutrients. They also bring balance to your hormones while helping reduce inflammation. Healthy fats have excellent skin benefits, as well—which is great if you have acne because of your condition. When it comes to ingredients that contain healthy fats which you can add to your recipes, look for:

- O Chia seeds

- O Flax seeds or flax meal

- O Almond butter (or other types of nut butter)

- O Salmon and other fatty fish

- O Avocados

- Lean proteins

On this diet, you should include healthy protein sources, too. And when it comes to protein, opt for lean sources. Protein is vital for your health as it provides you with energy while helping to build and maintain your muscle tissues. Some great examples of lean proteins are:

- O Eggs

- O Chicken breast

- O Tuna

- O Soy products

- Non-dairy milk

There are many different types of dairy products on the market. But when you're on the PCOS diet, it's recommended to reduce your intake of these foods. Since milk is one of the more common dairy products you can consume, going for non-dairy milk options allows you to enjoy this beverage while still being able to have other types of dairy, like cheese or yogurt, once in a while. You may also use non-dairy milk for your recipes if you want to make them dairy-free. Here are some examples of non-dairy milk products you can purchase from grocery stores:

- Rice milk

- Almond milk

- Soy milk

- Oat milk

- Coconut milk

- PCOS-friendly sweeteners

While it's recommended to avoid sugar in all forms, along with sugary foods, there are certain substitutes you can use when cooking, especially when making desserts. Some great examples of appropriate sweeteners are:

○ Coconut sugar

○ Manuka honey

These add a nice caramel-y flavor to your dishes and they offer some excellent health benefits, too. You can easily find these in your local supermarket, health food stores, or even in online shops.

• Snack items

While it's recommended to make your own snacks as part of your meal planning, you may also choose to purchase PCOS-diet friendly snacks to keep in your pantry. That way, if you're hungry and you've run out of prepped snacks, you can enjoy these healthy treats instead of grabbing something that doesn't work for your diet. Some examples are:

○ Organic goji berries

○ Trail mixes (with no added sugar)

○ Sweet potato chips

○ Dried fruits (with no added sugar)

○ Oatmeal cookies with raisins (with no added sugar)

When it comes to shopping for snacks, make it a habit to read the nutrition labels. This allows you to see if the snack items contain ingredients or caloric contents making them suitable—or not—for your diet. You can also find these snack items in supermarkets, specialty health stores, and online.

These are just some examples of healthy foods you can purchase for your new diet. Of course, the items you will include on your own shopping list will depend on the meals you have planned to make for the week. Later on, we will go through some healthy recipes you can start off with. Following recipes makes it easier for you to come up with a shopping list, as well as the quantities of foods you need to buy from supermarkets, health food stores, specialty stores, online stores, or other places where you do your food shopping.

Meal Planning on the PCOS Diet

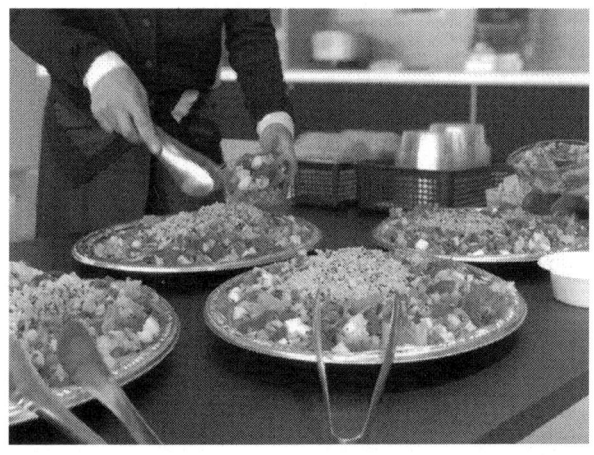

Meal planning is a beneficial aspect when following the PCOS diet because it helps you stick with your diet more effectively. Learning how to plan meals helps you become more organized and more aware of what you are eating. Also, meal planning aids you with creating a shopping list for when you need to buy food and ingredients at the store. If you want to manage your PCOS symptoms, shed some extra pounds, or even get pregnant, meal planning can go a long way toward helping you out.

Meal planning is a skill that gets easier the more you practice. It's a process that involves:

- Thinking of recipes

- Writing them down

- Checking your kitchen or pantry for any leftovers or ingredients you still have

- Making a list of ingredients you need

- Buying the required ingredients based on the list you have made

- Preparing the ingredients you have purchased

- Cooking all of the meals you have planned

It may seem quite overwhelming at first, but once you get the hang of it, you will realize that it's easy, fun, and saves you a lot of time and money in the long run. The great thing about meal planning is you have total control over the ingredients you include in your meals and in the portions of your meals.

Usually, you would plan your meals for one whole week, from breakfast to dinner and everything in between. To give you an idea, here's a sample plan for one day:

- **Breakfast:** Pumpkin Porridge

- **Lunch:** Stuffed Chicken Breasts

- **Snack:** Piña Colada Smoothie

- **Dinner:** Shrimp Salad with Broccoli and Cauliflower

- **Dessert:** Pastry Cream with Fruits

Simply think of the meals you normally consume throughout the day and create a list or a table as you're planning which recipes you will whip up. Here are some meal planning tips for you to remember:

- Set a schedule for your meal planning process. Include the planning process, shopping, preparation, and cooking. You can allocate one day for planning and shopping and one day for preparing and cooking.

- Come up with a rough draft of all the meals you want to have for the week. Then arrange them according to how long you can store the meals. For instance, meals with fresh ingredients like salads should be eaten sooner than meals that are fully cooked.

- Before planning, check your kitchen, pantry, and refrigerator. That way, you can incorporate any leftovers into your plans or think of recipes that include the ingredients you already have.

- When shopping for ingredients, make sure to stick with your list. This helps you save time and money, and ensures you stick to healthy options.

- Mix things up to keep your meals interesting. Find good combinations of sweet and savory dishes to make you feel full and satisfied throughout the day.

These days, meal planning is a lot easier because there are so many resources you can use. You can download meal planning templates online to keep you motivated, or search for recipes and other helpful tips to guide you.

Next up, we will be going through some healthy, easy, and tasty recipes you can start with. After you have practiced with these simple dishes, you can level up your game by searching for more complex recipes that include more ingredients!

Chapter 4: PCOS Diet Breakfast Recipes

Now that you know more about PCOS and how the PCOS diet can be beneficial to those suffering from this condition, let's go through some healthy, tasty, and simple recipes you can start making right now. When you suffer from PCOS, breakfast is one of the most important meals of the day—and this chapter focuses on nutritious breakfast recipes that will give you the energy you need to start your day off right.

No matter what your weight is, when you have this condition, you will also have some level of insulin resistance. Therefore, taking the necessary steps to maintain healthy blood sugar levels is a must. Consuming breakfast that contains the right amounts of macronutrients will help balance these levels. Also, eating a healthy meal at the start of your day will help you feel satisfied for a longer period of time. Before we go through the recipes, here are some useful PCOS diet breakfast tips for you to remember:

- When eating breakfast, slow down so you can get the most out of the meal. This allows you to make healthier food choices, and it also prevents you from feeling stressed.

- Avoid distractions—like using electronic gadgets or watching TV—while you have breakfast. This makes you more aware of what you are eating and how much you are eating.

- Pay attention to your body so you can observe how different kinds of food make you feel. This helps you determine which types of food or dishes satiate you so you feel full for longer periods of time.

- Pay attention to your body to determine if you have any food allergies or intolerances. Knowing which foods you are intolerant or allergic to helps you avoid them more effectively.

- Make sure your breakfast includes enough protein and healthy fats. These are very important when following the PCOS diet.

- It's also recommended to include fiber sources and anti-inflammatory foods into your breakfast meals. These types of food have a lot of health benefits that may improve PCOS symptoms.

- If you plan to include carbs, opt for low glycemic options. These have a less pronounced effect on your insulin and blood glucose levels.

- Find breakfast options that are both convenient and enjoyable. Convenient breakfast options prevent you from skipping meals, while enjoyable breakfast options ensure you feel happy and satisfied with what you have eaten.

- Prepare "back-up breakfasts" that you can eat whenever you are in a rush. That way, even if you overslept or you have too many things to do in the morning, you can still enjoy a filling and healthy breakfast.

There may be times when you want to skip breakfast. This is okay once in a while—as long as you don't eat more throughout the day to compensate. If you skip this important meal, make sure you continue eating the same portions for your lunch, snack, and dinner, as if you didn't skip breakfast. With that being said, let's move on to the recipes!

Stuffed Breakfast Bell Peppers

This first recipe is simple, savory, and will surely satisfy your cravings. The main ingredient—bell peppers—is great for PCOS, too. Like other brightly-colored veggies, bell peppers are rich in antioxidants, which help in the management of the condition. These antioxidants combat free radicals while reducing oxidative stress. When choosing peppers, opt for symmetrical ones with sides that are somewhat flat to make it easier to balance the peppers while you bake them.

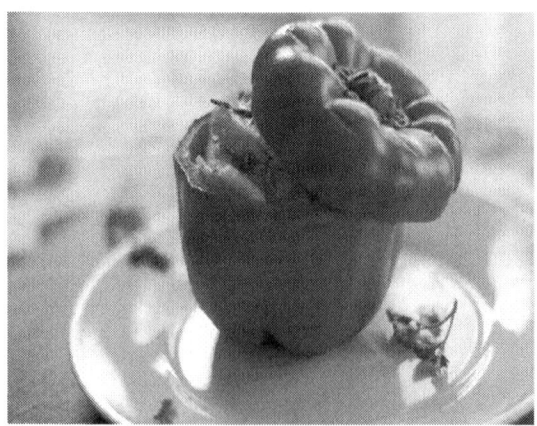

Nutritional Information for 1 stuffed bell pepper:

- Fat: 9.9 g

- Sodium: 0.73 g

- Potassium: 0.64 g

- Protein: 14.7 g

- Dietary Fiber: 2.7 g

- Carbs: 13.4 g

- Sugar: 2.2 g

Time: 45 minutes

Serving Size: 2 servings

Ingredients:

- ¼ tsp. cayenne pepper

- ½ tsp. black pepper

- ½ tsp. salt

- 1 cup broccoli (chopped into bite-sized pieces)

- 1 cup white mushrooms (roughly chopped)

- 2 medium-sized bell peppers

- 4 medium eggs

Directions:

1. Preheat your oven to 375°F and line a baking sheet with parchment paper.

2. In a bowl, combine the salt, pepper, cayenne, broccoli, mushrooms, and eggs.

3. Mix well and set aside.

4. Cut the peppers in half and remove the insides.

5. Divide the stuffing mixture equally and spoon it into each of the pepper halves.

6. Place the stuffed peppers on the baking sheet.

7. Place the baking sheet in the oven and cook the peppers for about 35 minutes.

8. Take the baking sheet out of the oven and serve while hot!

Blackberry Muffins

These moist and soft muffins are chock-full of healthy blackberries. Just like other berries, blackberries contain essential nutrients that help improve PCOS by boosting insulin resistance and combating inflammation. The berries provide the sweetness for the muffins, therefore, you don't need to add any sugar. Aside from being sugar-free, these low-carb muffins are gluten- and dairy-free, too. You can modify the recipe by replacing the blackberries with other kinds of berries.

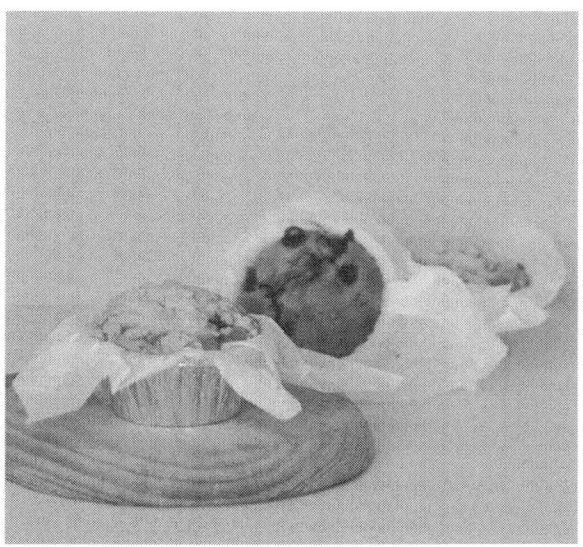

Nutritional Information for 1 muffin:

- Fat: 13.89 g

- Sodium: 0.05 g

- Protein: 4.53 g

- Fiber: 3.4 g

- Carbs: 6.76 g

- Sugar: 1.86 g

Time: 45 minutes

Serving Size: 12 muffins

Ingredients:

- ¼ tsp. baking soda

- ¼ tsp. salt

- 1 tsp. baking powder

- 1 tsp. vanilla extract

- 1 tbsp. coconut flour

- 2 tbsp. apple cider vinegar

- 2 tbsp. coconut oil (refined)

- ½ cup coconut cream (chilled)

- ½ cup sweetener of choice (powdered)

- 1 cup almond flour (blanched)

- 1 cup blueberries (frozen or fresh)

- 3 medium eggs

- Lemon zest

Directions:

1. Preheat your oven to 375°F and grease a muffin pan.

2. In a bowl, combine the coconut flour and blackberries, then mix well.

3. In a separate bowl, combine the baking soda, salt, baking powder, sweetener, almond flour, and lemon zest, then mix until well incorporated.

4. In another bowl, combine the vanilla extract, apple cider vinegar, coconut oil, coconut cream, and eggs, then mix until well incorporated.

5. Add the dry ingredient mixture and continue mixing to combine until you get a "spoonable" batter.

6. Fold the blackberries in gently until evenly incorporated.

7. Spoon the batter into the prepared muffin pan.

8. Place the pan in the oven and bake the muffins for about 35 minutes.

9. Take the pan out of the oven and allow the muffins to cool completely before you serve them.

Pumpkin Porridge

If you love eating oatmeal for breakfast, you'll surely love this recipe. Since oats are high in carbs, you'll need to find other kinds of recipes and substitutes to continue eating those heartwarming meals you're used to. Pumpkin is an excellent option to help manage the symptoms of PCOS and hormonal imbalances. It has a high fiber content, and it's rich in potassium, vitamin C, and other essential nutrients. Pumpkin is very versatile, too, as you can add it to various savory and sweet dishes.

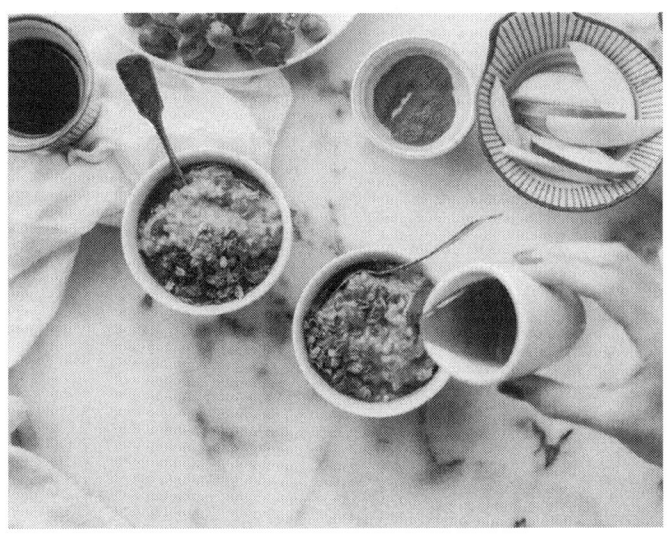

Nutritional Information for 1 bowl of porridge:

- Fat: 47 g

- Sodium: 0.01 g

- Potassium: 0.48 g

- Protein: 21.7 g

- Dietary Fiber: 6.3 g

- Carbohydrates: 27.2 g

- Sugar: 4.2 g

Time: 15 minutes

Serving Size: 1 serving

Ingredients:

- 1 tsp. cinnamon

- 1 tbsp. cashew butter

- 1 tbsp. ghee

- 2 tbsp. milk of choice (non-dairy)

- 3 tbsp. hemp seeds (hulled, shelled, ground)

- 3 tbsp. cashews (raw, ground)

- ⅓ cup pumpkin purée (fresh or canned)

- 1 tsp. sweetener of choice (powdered, optional)

- 1 tbsp. pumpkin seeds (optional)

Directions:

1. In a pot, heat the ghee over low heat.

2. Add all of the ingredients and mix well. You may add more milk to achieve the porridge consistency you desire. Add the sweetener, if desired.

3. Continue cooking on low heat until all of the ingredients have heated thoroughly.

4. Pour the porridge into a bowl and top with the pumpkin seeds, if desired. Serve while hot.

Breakfast Egg Muffins

These egg muffins are an excellent option for when you need to make a quick and easy breakfast. They contain healthy ingredients, with egg as the main focus. Eggs are another excellent food for PCOS sufferers. They are high in protein and contain other nutrients that help improve symptoms. Egg whites contain most of the protein, while the egg yolks contain omega-3 fatty acids, choline, thiamin, folate, iron, and different vitamins. If you plan to start meal prepping, you can also include these egg muffins because they store well, too.

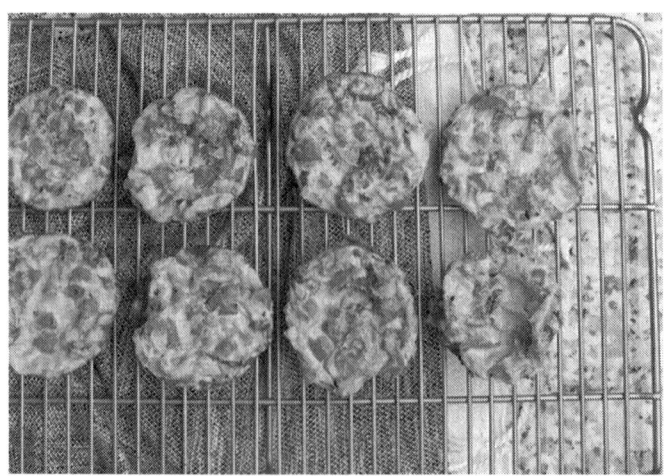

Nutritional Information for 1 egg muffin:

- Fat: 8.3 g

- Protein: 9.7 g

- Carbs: 2.1 g

Time: 30 minutes

Serving Size: 6 egg muffins

Ingredients:

- ¼ tsp. pepper (freshly ground)

- ½ cup kale (chopped)

- ½ lb. breakfast sausage (ground)

- 1 bell pepper (red, diced)

- 1 bell pepper (yellow, diced)

- 9 large eggs

Directions:

1. Preheat your oven to 350°F and grease a muffin pan.

2. In a skillet, brown the ground sausage over medium heat. Transfer to a bowl without the grease.

75

3. Add the kale, peppers, eggs, and pepper to the bowl, then whisk until well combined.

4. Spoon the mixture into the prepared muffin pan.

5. Place the pan in the oven and bake the egg muffins for 20 to 25 minutes.

6. Take the muffin pan out of the oven and allow the egg muffins to cool before removing and serving.

Quinoa Fritters

These fritters are crunchy, savory, and oh-so-healthy—they even come with a tasty dipping sauce that will keep you coming back for more. Quinoa is now considered a superfood because it has a lovely texture, it's highly versatile, and it has an excellent nutrition profile. Quinoa also provides a delicious nutty taste and is chock-full of amino acids. This complete protein is great for PCOS as well, so you may want to use it in other dishes. Technically, quinoa is a fruit, not a grain, and it's an excellent alternative to rice or couscous which are high in carbs.

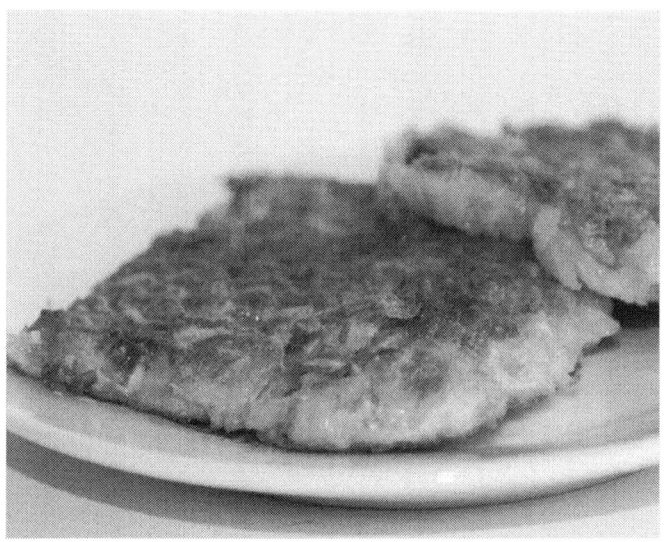

Nutritional Information for 1 fritter:

- Fat: 53 g

- Sodium: 0.84 g

- Protein: 17 g

- Fiber: 8 g

- Carbs: 38 g

- Sugar: 5 g

Time: 25 minutes

Serving Size: 6 fritters (average size)

Ingredients for the quinoa fritters:

- 1 tbsp. chives (chopped)

- 1 tbsp. coriander (chopped)

- 3 tbsp. coconut oil

- ¼ cup almond meal

- 1 cup quinoa (cooked)

- 1 medium-sized carrot (grated)

- 1 small onion (finely chopped)

- 3 medium-sized eggs

- Pepper

- Salt

Ingredients for the garlic aioli dip:

- ¼ tsp. sea salt

- 1 tbsp. Dijon mustard

- 2 tbsp. lemon juice

- 2 tbsp. olive oil

- ½ cup cashews or almonds (blanched, soaked for at least 4 hours)

- ½ cup water

- 2 garlic cloves (minced)

Directions:

1. In a bowl, combine all of the fritter ingredients and mix well.

2. In a frying pan, heat 3 tablespoons of coconut oil over medium heat.

3. Use a soup spoon to scoop the fritter mixture and gently place into the frying pan. Using the same

spoon, flatten the fritters a bit by gently pressing down on them.

4. Cook the quinoa fritters for a couple of minutes, flip, and continue cooking until they turn golden.

5. Take the quinoa fritters out of the frying pan and allow the excess oil to drain onto a paper towel.

6. Repeat the last three steps until you have used up all of the quinoa fritter mixture. Add coconut oil to the pan as needed.

7. In a blender, combine all of the garlic aioli dip ingredients except for the water.

8. Blend on high until well incorporated.

9. Add the water gradually, then continue blending until you achieve a creamy consistency.

10. Transfer the dipping sauce into a small bowl and serve with the hot quinoa fritters.

Chapter 5: PCOS Diet Lunch Recipes

When it comes to lunch and dinner recipes, there are so many options to choose from. These versatile recipes are easy, healthy, and scrumptious, too. You can even have these dishes for dinner, just make sure that you count your macros before eating a fuller or heavier dinner. Part of the PCOS diet involves making sure that you take in enough nutrients each day. This means that you have to get all the fats, proteins, carbs, and other nutrients you need all day from the meals you prepare for yourself.

Zucchini Lasagna

This tasty, low-carb recipe makes use of zucchini for the noodles instead of pasta, which is high in carbs. Consuming a lot of whole foods such as zucchini will help you better manage your condition. A whole-food PCOS diet has anti-inflammatory effects and helps nourish your body as needed. As with other veggies, zucchini contains fiber to help improve your digestive processes. Plus, this vegetable has a wonderful texture, making it the perfect substitution for lasagna noodles. This dish is sugar-, grain-, and gluten-free, but full of wonderful flavors from the combination of ingredients.

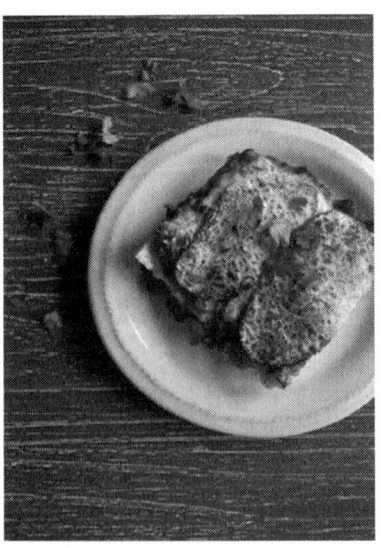

Nutritional Information for 1 slice of lasagna:

- Fat: 32.2 g

- Sodium: 0.53 g

- Potassium: 0.73 g

- Protein: 16.58 g

- Fiber: 2.8 g

- Carbs: 11.36 g

- Sugar: 2.62 g

Time: 1 hour and 10 minutes

Serving Size: 6 servings

Ingredients for the lasagna:

- ¼ cup black olives

- ½ cup mozzarella cheese (shredded)

- ¾ cup spinach (boiled)

- 2 cups mascarpone

- 1 ½ eggs (hard-boiled)

- 2 ½ zucchinis (choose straight and fat pieces, sliced into strips)

Ingredients for the meat sauce:

- ½ tsp. black pepper
- ½ tsp. salt
- ½ tbsp. basil
- ½ tbsp. garlic powder
- ½ tbsp. olive oil
- ½ tbsp. oregano
- ½ tbsp. parsley
- 1 tbsp. tomato paste
- ½ cup brown mushrooms (chopped)
- ½ cup water
- 1 ½ cups tomatoes (crushed)
- ½ lb. ground beef
- ¼ onion (chopped)
- 1 bay leaf
- 1 ½ garlic cloves
- 2 ½ zucchini (cores, chopped)

Directions:

1. If you haven't sliced the zucchinis yet, start by doing this. Cut off the ends of the zucchinis before cutting them into strips. Use a vegetable peeler to slice the strips all the way to the core. Set aside the zucchini slices and the zucchini cores.

2. In a pot, add a tablespoon of olive oil and cook the garlic and onions for about one minute over medium heat.

3. Add the beef, then continue cooking until the meat starts browning.

4. Add the zucchini cores and mushrooms, then continue cooking to soften.

5. Add the tomato paste, tomatoes, and all the spices, then stir well.

6. Turn down the heat to medium-low and allow the sauce to simmer for about 20 minutes. Stir occasionally to prevent the sauce from sticking to the bottom of your pot.

7. Once ready, take the sauce off the heat and set aside.

8. Preheat your oven to 400°F and grease a baking dish.

9. Spoon a layer of sauce into the bottom of the baking dish and top with zucchini noodles. Spoon another layer of sauce and top with more zucchini noodles.

10. Then, top with half of the mascarpone, half of the spinach, and more zucchini noodles.

11. Top with more sauce, boiled eggs, and zucchini noodles. Finally, top with half of the mascarpone, half of the spinach, the black olives, more sauce, and zucchini noodles.

12. For the top, spread a final layer of meat sauce then cover with the mozzarella cheese.

13. Place the baking dish in the oven and bake the lasagna for about 30 minutes.

14. Take the baking dish out of the oven and allow to cool before slicing and serving.

Mediterranean-Style Tuna Salad

Most of the time, tuna salad recipes call for a lot of mayonnaise. Unfortunately, commercial mayonnaise products contain a lot of PCOS-unfriendly ingredients. While you have the option to make your own mayonnaise for tuna salad, you could also try this unique twist on the classic salad. Tuna is an oily fish that contains good amounts of fatty acids and proteins. This makes it an ideal addition to your diet. This salad also contains other healthy ingredients that are perfect for your new diet—and for improving PCOS symptoms. Eat this salad on its own, with crackers, on a sandwich with low-carb bread, and more.

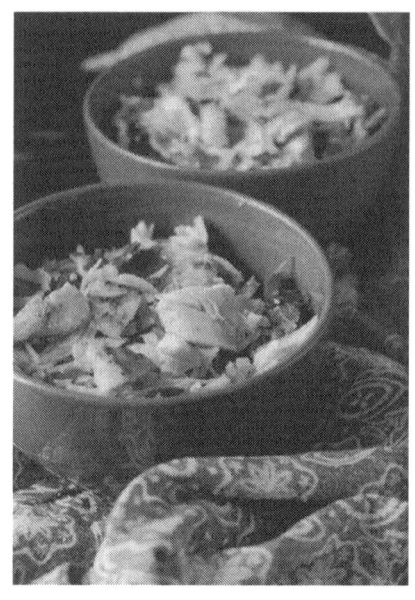

Nutritional Information for 1 serving of tuna salad:

- Fat: 25 g

- Sodium: 0.62 g

- Protein: 20 g

- Dietary Fiber: 6 g

- Carbs: 14 g

- Sugar: 3 g

Time: 5 minutes

Serving Size: 2 servings

Ingredients:

- 2 tbsp. basil leaves (fresh, slivered)
- 3 tbsp. olive oil
- ¼ cup parsley (fresh, chopped)
- ½ cup artichoke hearts (diced)
- ½ cup kalamata olives (pitted, chopped)
- ¾ cup tuna (canned)
- 1 bell pepper (roasted, chopped)
- 1 lemon (juiced)
- Black pepper
- Salt

Directions:

1. In a bowl, combine all of the ingredients. Season with salt and pepper then toss lightly until well combined.

2. Place in the refrigerator to chill.

3. Serve on keto bread, lettuce leaves, or your choice of sides.

Stuffed Chicken Breasts

This is a delicious gluten- and starch-free lunch that you can have ready in half an hour. Here, you will stuff the chicken breasts with healthy ingredients, one of which is spinach. This dark and leafy green contains various nutrients, including vitamin B6, vitamin C, and vitamin K. All of these vitamins are beneficial for PCOS because they help reduce inflammation. The great thing about this recipe is you can choose other greens to replace spinach since most dark, leafy greens contain similar nutrients.

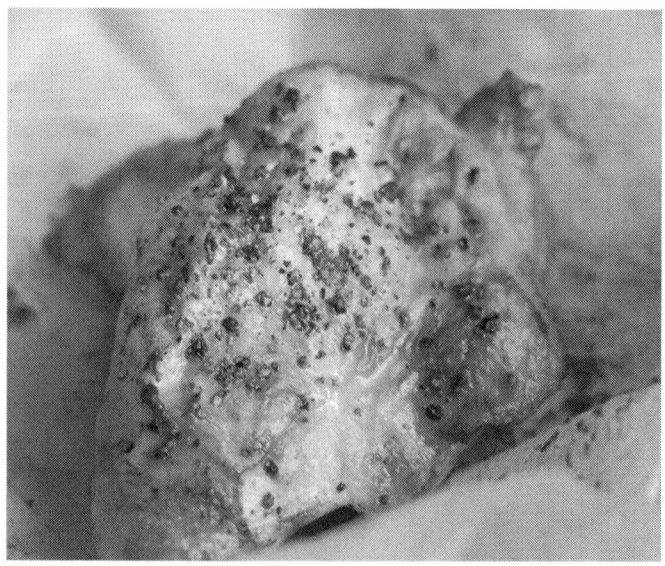

Nutritional Information for 1 serving:

- Fat: 25.19 g

- Sodium: 1.28 g

- Potassium: 0.28 g

- Protein: 55.41 g

- Fiber: 1.2 g

- Carbs: 5.62 g

- Sugar: 2.25 g

Time: 30 minutes

Serving Size: 4 servings

Ingredients:

- ½ tsp. black pepper

- ½ tsp. salt

- ½ tsp. xanthan gum

- 1 tbsp. olive oil

- ¼ cup parsley (fresh, chopped)

- ½ cup heavy cream

- ⅔ cup spinach (wilted)

- ¾ cup feta cheese

- 2 cups chicken broth

- 2 garlic cloves (minced)

- 3 chicken breasts (boneless, skinless)

Directions:

1. Slice the chicken breasts lengthwise, but not all the way. Open the halves, cover with plastic food wrap, and use a meat pounder to tenderize the chicken breasts and flatten them out.

2. Peel the plastic food wrap off and season the chicken breasts with salt and pepper.

3. In a bowl, combine the spinach, feta cheese, and garlic, then mix well. Divide the mixture into three equal portions.

4. Spoon the mixture into the center of each chicken breast, roll them up, and secure them with toothpicks.

5. In a skillet, warm olive oil over medium heat.

6. Add the stuffed chicken breasts and cook for about 4 to 5 minutes on each side.

7. Pour the chicken broth into the skillet, turn the heat down to medium-low, and allow to simmer for about 10 minutes. After 5 minutes, flip the stuffed chicken breasts over.

8. Transfer the stuffed chicken breasts to a chopping board and carefully remove the toothpicks.

9. Add the cream to the chicken broth and bring to a boil.

10. Once the mixture boils, add the xanthan gum and a pinch of black pepper, then whisk vigorously to thicken the sauce.

11. When the sauce is thick enough, place the stuffed chicken breasts back into the skillet. Sprinkle with fresh parsley and serve while hot.

Gazpacho Soup

This soup is super healthy as it calls for unpeeled cucumber, tomatoes, and other fresh ingredients to maximize its health benefits. Tomatoes contain lycopene, a type of carotenoid that helps combat PCOS, cancer, and heart disease. Since the body doesn't produce this carotenoid naturally, you must consume a lot of foods that are rich in it—like tomatoes. This recipe also contains red onions, which are chock-full of flavonoids. Aside from being really healthy, this cold soup is easy to make, too!

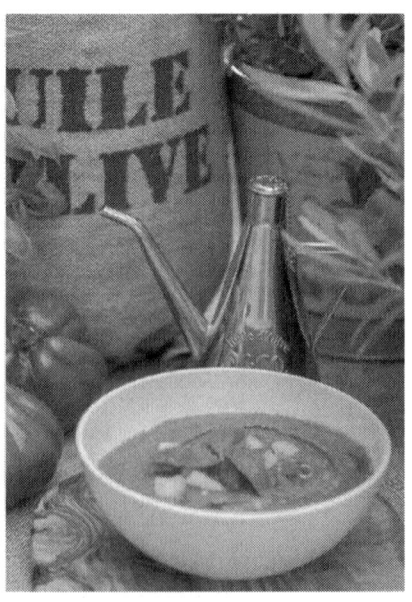

Nutritional Information for 1 bowl of soup:

- Fat: 15 g
- Sodium: 0.62 g
- Protein: 5 g
- Fiber: 6 g
- Carbs: 30 g

Time: 30 minutes

Serving Size: 3 servings

Ingredients:

- 1 tsp. black pepper
- 1 tsp. salt
- 1 tbsp. lemon juice
- 3 tbsp. balsamic vinegar
- 4 tbsp. olive oil
- 1 medium-sized cucumber
- 1 medium-sized red onion
- 1 slice of whole-wheat bread
- 2 bell peppers (any color)

- 2 garlic cloves

- 8 medium-sized tomatoes (ripe)

- Fresh microgreens or herbs (for garnishing)

Directions:

1. Wash the tomatoes, cut them into quarters, and remove the bases of the stems.

2. Cut the cucumber, onion, garlic, and bell peppers roughly.

3. Put all of the vegetables in a food processor, then blend well.

4. Tear the slice of bread into chunks and add to the food processor.

5. Allow the mixture to sit for about 20 minutes so the bread softens as it absorbs the liquid.

6. Add the lemon juice, olive oil, and vinegar to the mixture and continue processing until all ingredients have liquefied.

7. Season with salt and pepper, then process for a few more seconds.

8. Pour the soup into a bowl, cover with a lid, and place in the refrigerator overnight.

9. Serve the gazpacho soup chilled and garnish with microgreens or herbs.

Cauliflower Stuffing

These days, there are so many recipes that incorporate cauliflower. It's used as an alternative to rice, as the main ingredient for bread, and as a replacement for other high-carb food items. In this recipe, cauliflower also stars as the main ingredient. This cruciferous veggie ranks low on the glycemic index. The nutrient profile of this vegetable makes it filling and the perfect choice for those who want to lose weight and manage PCOS symptoms. This is another simple recipe that's starch-, grain-, gluten-, and dairy-free.

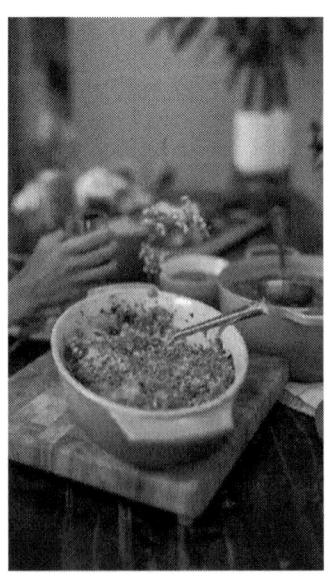

Nutritional Information for 1 serving:

- Fat: 13.24 g

- Sodium: 0.89 g

- Potassium: 0.85 g

- Protein: 19.44 g

- Fiber: 5 g

- Carbs: 13.7 g

- Sugar: 6.06 g

Time: 55 minutes

Serving Size: 4 servings

Ingredients:

- ½ tsp. black pepper

- ¾ tsp. salt

- ½ tbsp. sage (chopped)

- ½ tbsp. thyme (chopped)

- 2 tbsp. butter

- ¼ cup parsley (fresh, chopped)

- ½ cup chicken bone broth

- ½ lb. ground chicken

- ¼ onion (chopped)

- 1 garlic clove (minced)

- 1 large cauliflower (cut into florets)

- 1 small carrot (chopped)

- 2 celery sticks (chopped)

- 5 brown mushrooms (sliced)

Directions:

1. In a pot, add the butter and melt over low heat.

2. Add the onion, celery, garlic, and carrot, then cook for about 15 minutes until the onions start caramelizing and the carrot pieces have softened.

3. Add the ground chicken and mix to break down any chunks.

4. Add all of the spices and the mushrooms and continue cooking to soften the mushrooms.

5. Add the cauliflower and cook for about 3 more minutes.

6. Pour in the chicken bone broth, cover, and allow to steam for about 3 minutes.

7. Remove the lid and continue cooking until the broth has evaporated completely.

8. Transfer the stuffing to a bowl and serve while hot.

Chapter 6: PCOS Diet Dinner Recipes

While many people tend to skip dinner when they are dieting in an attempt to lose more weight, you don't have to do this. It's all about learning how to spread out your food intake—and macros—throughout the day. Since you will be restricting certain foods from your diet, you must still make sure that you are eating enough nutrients each day. This ensures that you remain healthy even while you are losing weight and enjoying all the other benefits of the PCOS diet. When planning your meals, take note of the total calorie counts as well as the amount of fat, protein, and carbs in each meal you are eating. This allows you to make calculations and ensure you're not exceeding or eating less than what is required.

Honey and Sesame Chicken

This easy recipe tastes just like the popular takeout dish—and since it's healthier, it's even better! It incorporates natural ingredients that fit right into your PCOS diet and are beneficial to your overall health. The main ingredient of this dish—chicken breast—is a high-protein, low-fat food item. It contains vitamin B3, vitamin B6, and other B vitamins. In particular, vitamin B6 is essential for managing PCOS, as it's an excellent hormone regulator and fertility booster. If you want to maintain a clean diet, opt for organic chicken to reduce the risk of ingesting harmful toxins.

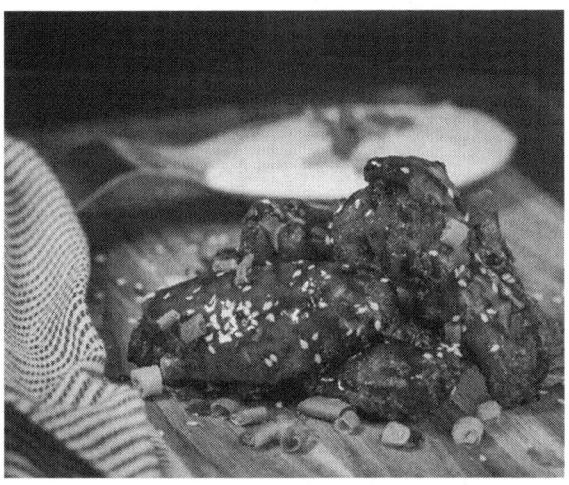

Nutritional Information for 1 serving:

- Fat: 23 g

- Protein: 35 g

- Fiber: 1 g

- Carbs: 21 g

- Sugar: 10 g

Time: 30 minutes

Serving Size: 4 servings

Ingredients for the chicken:

- ¼ tsp. sea salt

- ½ tsp. black pepper

- 2 tbsp. arrowroot powder

- 3 tbsp. coconut oil

- 2 cups broccoli (cut into florets)

- 1 ½ lbs. chicken breast (boneless, skinless)

- 1 large egg

Ingredients for the sauce:

- ¼ tsp. sea salt
- ½ tsp. red pepper flakes (crushed)
- 1 tbsp. toasted sesame oil
- 1 ½ tbsp. arrowroot powder
- 2 tbsp. water
- 3 tbsp. white wine vinegar
- ¼ cup honey
- ¼ cup sesame seeds
- ⅓ cup coconut aminos
- 1 piece of ginger (2 inches, fresh, grated)

Directions:

1. Cut the chicken breasts into bite-sized pieces and set aside.

2. In a bowl, combine the arrowroot powder, pepper, salt, and eggs, then whisk until smooth.

3. Add the chicken into the mixture and toss until all pieces are evenly coated.

4. In a separate bowl, combine all of the sauce ingredients and whisk together until there are no more clumps left.

5. In a skillet, warm the coconut oil over medium-high heat.

6. Add the chicken and cook for about 2 minutes each side until crispy, golden, and almost cooked through.

7. After frying all of the pieces of chicken, add the remaining mixture into the skillet, along with all of the chicken pieces. Also, add the broccoli.

8. Toss all of the ingredients lightly for a couple of minutes for everything to become crispy.

9. Add the sauce and continue tossing.

10. Transfer the chicken to a serving bowl and serve while hot.

Grain Bowl

The great thing about grain bowls is that they are healthy, tasty, versatile, and completely customizable. This recipe is just one example of a healthy grain bowl suitable for the PCOS diet. Choosing the right ingredients for your grain bowl provides you with a satisfying meal filled with antioxidants and other essential nutrients. One such ingredient in this recipe is chickpeas. As with other legumes, chickpeas are high in fiber and other essential minerals. Chickpeas are protein-rich, too, which means that they will fill you up for a longer time. This ingredient is also associated with lower insulin and blood sugar levels. And they're tasty, too!

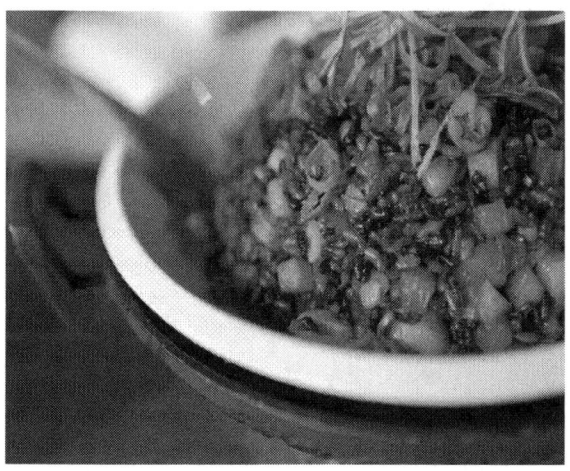

Nutritional Information for 1 bowl:

- Fat: 26 g
- Sodium: 0.43 g
- Protein: 15 g
- Fiber: 8 g
- Carbs: 46 g

Time: 15 minutes

Serving Size: 1 serving

Ingredients:

- 1 tbsp. olive oil
- 1 tbsp. walnut pesto
- 1 tbsp. pine nuts
- ¼ cup chickpeas (canned or cooked)
- ¼ cup quinoa (cooked)
- 1 cup zucchini (spiralized)
- 1 ½ cups broccoli (florets)
- black pepper
- salt

Directions:

1. Preheat your oven to 350°F and grease a baking sheet.

2. Place the broccoli on the baking sheet, drizzle with olive oil, then season with salt and pepper. Toss lightly to coat all the florets evenly.

3. Place the baking sheet in the oven and roast the broccoli florets for about 30 minutes.

4. Take the baking sheet out of the oven and set the broccoli florets aside.

5. In a bowl, combine the pesto, zucchini, and quinoa. Toss lightly, and allow to sit for 3 to 5 minutes.

6. Add the roasted broccoli florets, pine nuts, and chickpeas. Add more salt and pepper as needed, then serve immediately.

Shrimp Salad with Broccoli and Cauliflower

This is a healthy, creamy low-carb dish that will surely fill your tummy and satisfy your cravings. It's made with nutritious ingredients and has a combination of flavors that is totally irresistible! What makes this salad special is that it contains shrimp—a healthy type of seafood that offers a number of health benefits such as weight management, a reduced risk of cardiovascular disease, and improved brain and bone health. It also helps lower inflammation, which is great when you suffer from PCOS. With all these health benefits, you should keep eating shrimp as part of your healing PCOS diet.

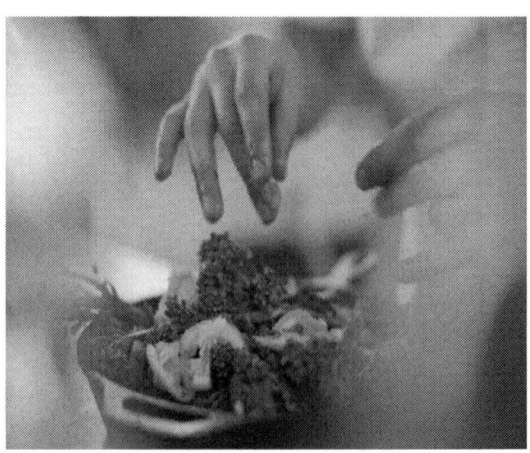

Nutritional Information for 1 serving:

- Fat: 22.6 g
- Sodium: 0.97 g
- Potassium: 0.77 g
- Protein: 25.15 g
- Fiber: 5.4 g
- Carbs: 14.68 g
- Sugar: 4.92 g

Time: 15 minutes

Serving Size: 4 servings

Ingredients:

- ½ tsp. black pepper
- ½ tsp. salt
- 2 tsp. olive oil
- 1 tbsp. oregano
- 6 tbsp. mayonnaise
- ¼ cup cheddar cheese (grated)
- 1 ¼ cups shrimp
- 1 ¾ cups broccoli (cut into florets)

- 1 ¾ cups cauliflower (cut into florets)

- ¼ red onion (diced)

- 1 large tomato (diced)

- 3 garlic cloves (minced)

Directions:

1. In a pot, bring water to a boil on medium heat.

2. Add the broccoli and cauliflower florets and cook for 4 to 5 minutes, until tender. Drain then set aside to cool completely.

3. In a frying pan, add the olive oil and garlic, then cook over medium heat for about 1 minute.

4. Add the shrimps and sauté until cooked completely. Transfer to a bowl and set aside to cool.

5. In a bowl, combine all of the ingredients and mix well. Spoon into serving bowls and serve.

Tuna Melt

This unique tuna melt is light on the mayonnaise and topped with fresh tomato slices. We've already discussed how beneficial tuna and tomato are for your health when you suffer from PCOS. This particular recipe also includes shredded cheese. While it's recommended for PCOS sufferers to limit dairy intake, having a few servings occasionally may be helpful, especially since dairy contains calcium. If your other meals of the day don't include any dairy products, you can enjoy this tuna melt for dinner guilt-free!

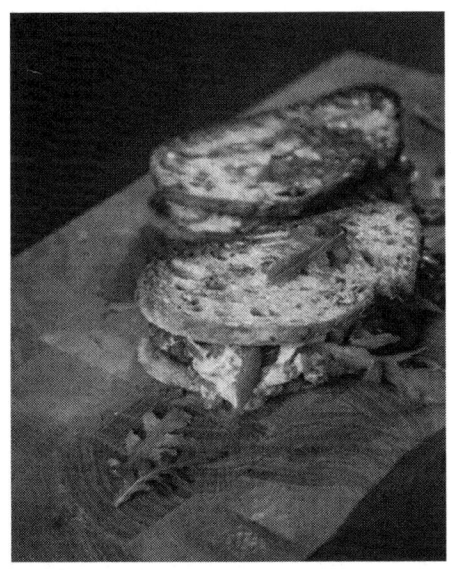

Nutritional Information for 1 tuna melt:

- Fat: 8 g
- Sodium: 0.46 g
- Potassium: 0.33 g
- Protein: 16 g
- Fiber: 3 g
- Carbs: 17 g
- Sugar: 3 g

Time: 15 minutes

Serving Size: 4 servings

Ingredients:

- ⅛ tsp. salt
- 1 tbsp. lemon juice
- 1 tbsp. parsley (minced)
- 2 tbsp. mayonnaise
- ½ cup sharp cheddar cheese (shredded)
- 1 ¼ cup tuna (canned, drained)
- 1 medium-sized shallot (minced)
- 2 medium-sized tomatoes (sliced)

- 4 slices of whole-wheat bread (toasted)
- Black pepper
- Hot sauce (optional)

Directions:

1. Preheat your oven to 350°F and grease a baking sheet.

2. In a bowl, combine the salt, lemon juice, parsley, mayonnaise, shallot, pepper, tuna, and hot sauce (if desired), then mix well.

3. Divide the mixture evenly by spreading it on top of each slice of toasted bread.

4. Top with slices of tomato and sprinkle with cheese.

5. Place the tuna melt slices on the prepared baking sheet.

6. Place the baking sheet in the oven and broil the tuna melt slices for 3 to 5 minutes, until the cheese starts bubbling.

7. Take the baking sheet out of the oven and allow the tuna melt slices to cool down slightly before serving.

Turkey with Pomegranate Glaze and Roasted Fennel

Pairing turkey cutlets with a rich pomegranate sauce and roasted fennel makes for a simple but elegant meal. You can even garnish with fresh pomegranate seeds to further elevate this dish. Beyond the appearance, the ingredients included in this dish make it suitable for your diet and beneficial for PCOS, as well. Turkey is an excellent source of protein, which will fill you up for a longer time. Pomegranates are healthy, too, because they contain quercetin, lycopene, and ellagic acid, all of which help lower the lipid profile. This is a specific benefit that applies to those suffering from PCOS.

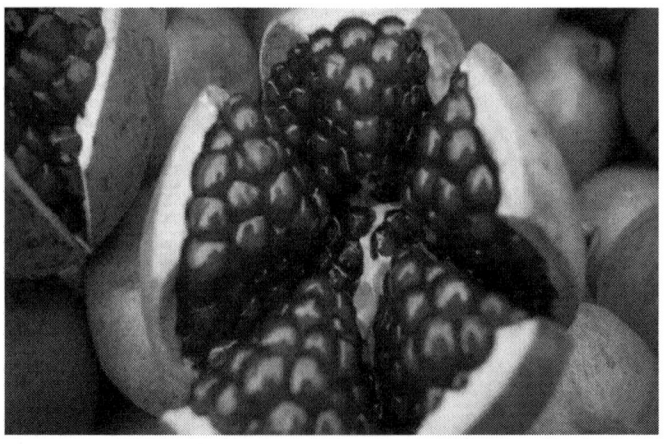

Nutritional Information for 1 serving:

- Fat: 7 g

- Sodium: 0.5 g

- Potassium: 1.46 g

- Protein: 31 g

- Fiber: 7 g

- Carbs: 26 g

- Sugar: 17 g

Time: 30 minutes

Serving Size: 4 servings

Ingredients:

- ½ tsp. thyme (fresh, chopped)

- ¾ tsp. pepper (freshly ground)

- 1 tsp. corn starch

- 1 tsp. kosher salt

- 5 tsp. canola oil

- ¼ cup chicken broth (reduced sodium)

- 1 cup pomegranate juice

- 1 lb. turkey cutlets (cut into slices with ¼-inch thickness)

- 4 medium-sized fennel bulbs (cored, sliced thickly)

Directions:

1. Preheat your oven to 450°F and grease a baking sheet.

2. In a bowl, combine the thyme, 3 teaspoons of canola oil, ¼ teaspoon of salt, ¼ teaspoon of pepper, and the fennel bulbs, then toss lightly.

3. Spread the coated fennel bulb slices on the baking sheet.

4. Place the baking sheet in the oven and roast the fennel bulb slices for about 25 minutes, until golden and tender. Stir the fennel bulb slices twice while roasting.

5. Use the remaining salt and pepper to season the turkey cutlets.

6. In a skillet, warm 2 teaspoons of canola oil over medium-high heat.

7. Add the turkey slices and cook for 1 to 3 minutes on each side, until browned.

8. Transfer the cooked turkey slices to a plate.

9. In the same skillet, add the pomegranate juice and a sprig of thyme, then bring the liquid to a boil. Stir frequently for 5 to 10 minutes, until the liquid has reduced to ¼ cup.

10. Remove the sprig of thyme.

11. In a bowl, combine the chicken broth and cornstarch, then mix well.

12. Add to the skillet and continue cooking to thicken for about 15 seconds, stirring constantly.

13. Lower the heat to medium and add the cooked turkey to the skillet for about 1 more minute.

14. Once done, transfer the glazed turkey slices to serving plates and top with roasted fennel. Serve while hot.

Chapter 7: PCOS Diet Dessert Recipes

One of the most effective ways you can overcome PCOS is by avoiding sugar in all forms, including sugary foods. When you follow the PCOS diet, you are advised to avoid sugar, or limit your sugar intake. For a lot of people, both cases are extremely difficult. But the good news is, with the proper knowledge of appropriate sweeteners and sugar substitutes, you can continue eating yummy desserts while following this special diet—and trying to improve your condition.

If you love desserts and sugary sweets, here are some tips to help you out. You don't have to quit cold-turkey—all you have to do is know what types of sweet treats you can have and how to make them. Consider these pointers:

- There are two main types of sugars—fructose and glucose. Between these two, glucose is the better option, because fructose promotes fat storage and has a negative impact on your fertility. If you have to choose a sweetener, it's better to go for those which are glucose-based.

- Some examples of glucose-based sweeteners you can use for your recipes are corn syrup, dextrose, and brown rice syrup. Conversely, some examples of fructose-based sweeteners you must avoid include yacon syrup, maple syrup, and more.

- Include a lot of protein and healthy fats into your recipes to counter the harmful effects of glucose in your body. With such nutrients, the glucose you consume will be absorbed by your body more gradually which, in turn, leads to a steadier rise in blood sugar levels.

- There are a lot of plant-based sweeteners you can use, as well. The great thing about these is that a lot of them are fructose- and glucose-free.

- Gradually wean yourself off sweets. Whether you are a sweet-treat monster or you only enjoy sweets occasionally, reducing the amount of sugar you eat or add to your recipes makes the transition much easier.

With these simple tips in mind, you may find that giving up your sweet cravings isn't that difficult. Don't be too hard on yourself. If you're craving something sweet, whip up a healthy dessert instead of restricting yourself and allowing your craving to go unsatisfied. Following are some easy recipes to start you off.

Choco-Avocado Mousse

This mousse is thick, creamy, and oh-so-easy. It's the ultimate dessert to satisfy your sweet tooth and it's packed with essential nutrients, too. One of the main ingredients of this recipe is avocado— a very popular superfood. It's rich in saturated fat, essential fatty acids, and other vitamins and minerals that help reduce inflammation, improve the health of your skin, and promote healthy functions of the immune and endocrine systems. You can make this choco-avocado mousse in a matter of minutes, and one bite will get you hooked.

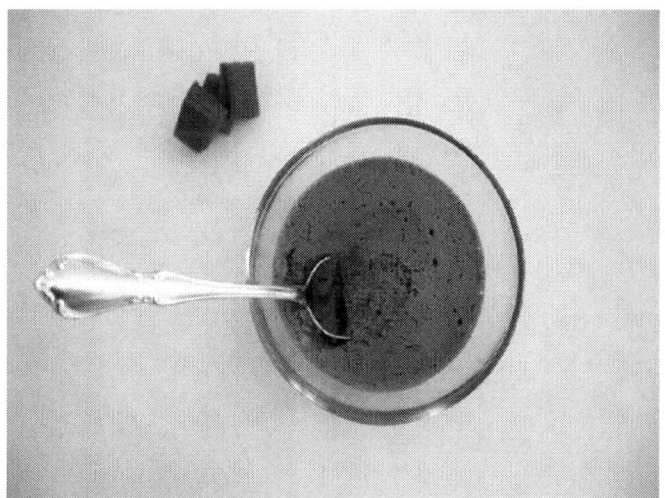

Nutritional Information for 1 serving:

- Fat: 14 g

- Protein: 2.8 g

- Fiber: 6.7 g

- Carbs: 10.5 g

- Sugar: 0.8 g

Time: 5 minutes

Serving Size: 6 servings

Ingredients:

- ½ tsp. vanilla extract

- 1 tsp. cinnamon

- ½ cup cocoa powder (unsweetened)

- ½ cup coconut cream

- ½ cup sweetener (powdered)

- 2 large avocados (pitted, peeled)

- Nutmeg

- Sea salt

Directions:

1. In a food processor, add all of the measured ingredients plus a pinch of nutmeg and a pinch of salt.

2. Blend everything together until you achieve a smooth and creamy consistency.

3. Divide the mousse between six serving bowls or glasses and place in the refrigerator to chill before serving.

Lemon Fat Bombs

These healthy fat bombs are tasty, healthy, and perfectly tart. These serve as the perfect ending to any kind of meal. They're delicious, filling, and contain lemons—a simple yet healthy fruit. Lemons are nourishing and they offer some incredible healing properties, too. They help with hormonal balance, promote efficient digestion, have a positive effect on the regulation of glucose levels, and may even help improve insulin resistance. After whipping up a batch of these tasty fat bombs, you can store them in your refrigerator for whenever you need a dessert with a kick.

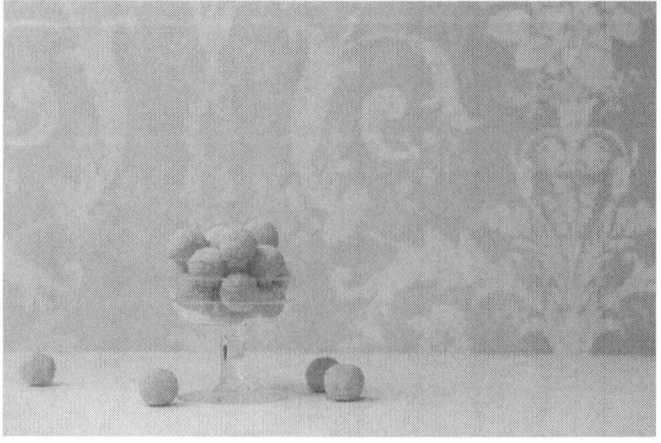

Nutritional Information for 1 fat bomb:

- Fat: 15 g
- Protein: 2.3 g
- Dietary fiber: 1.4 g
- Carbs: 5.7 g

Time: 1 hour

Serving Size: 30 fat bombs (depending on the size)

Ingredients:

- ¼ cup coconut flour
- ⅓ cup coconut (shredded)
- ½ cup coconut butter
- 1 cup coconut oil
- 1 large lemon (zest)
- 2 cups cashews (raw, soaked for at least 2 hours or boiled for about 12 minutes)
- 2 large lemons (juiced)
- Sweetener (powdered)
- Pink Himalayan salt

Directions:

1. In a food processor, combine all of the measured ingredients plus a pinch of sweetener and a pinch of salt, then pulse until everything is well-combined.

2. Transfer the mixture to a bowl, then place in your freezer for 30 to 40 minutes.

3. Take the mixture out of the freezer and use your hands to form small balls. Place the fat bombs on a parchment-lined cookie sheet.

4. Place the cookie sheet into your freezer for about 20 more minutes to set.

5. Once solid, transfer the fat bombs into an airtight container and store in the refrigerator until ready to serve.

Dark Chocolate Bark with Chickpeas

This chocolate bark is a unique dessert that you will surely love. It's salty, sweet, soft, and has a slight crunch to it. This is a simple recipe that only requires five ingredients, one of which is dark chocolate. According to research, dark chocolate helps improve the regulation of glucose, increase circulation, reduce hypertension, and may even promote weight loss. Finishing off your meal with this dark chocolate bark will promote satiety, soothe your nerves, and improve your mood. This is an excellent dessert option for PCOS sufferers who love chocolate.

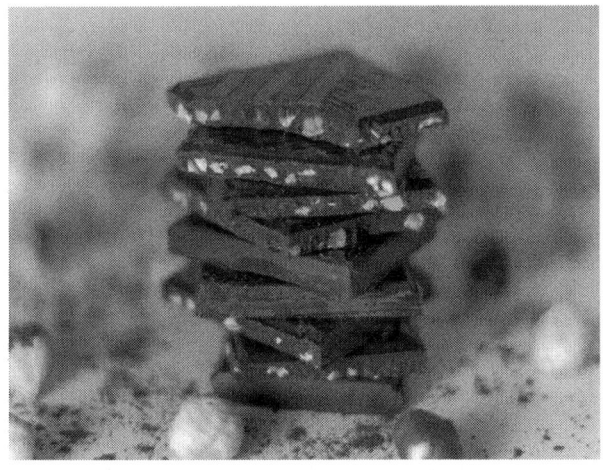

Nutritional Information for 1 serving:

- Fat: 10 g

- Protein: 3 g

- Carbs: 16 g

Time: 20 minutes

Serving Size: 1 batch (about 12 servings)

Ingredients:

- 1 tbsp. cinnamon (ground)

- 2 tbsp. coconut oil

- 1 cup dark chocolate chips (sugar-free, dairy-free)

- 2 ½ cups chickpeas

- Sea salt

Directions:

1. Preheat your oven to 400°F and line a baking sheet with parchment paper.

2. Rinse the chickpeas and spread evenly on the baking sheet.

3. Place the baking sheet in the oven and bake the chickpeas for 8 to 10 minutes, until completely dry.

4. Take the baking sheet out of the oven and transfer the chickpeas to a bowl.

5. Add the cinnamon and coconut oil and mix until all the chickpeas are evenly coated.

6. Pour the chickpeas back onto the baking sheet and lightly sprinkle with sea salt.

7. Place the baking sheet back into the oven and continue roasting the chickpeas for about 40 more minutes. Every 15 minutes, shake the baking sheet to ensure that the chickpeas roast evenly.

8. Take the baking sheet out of the oven and allow the chickpeas to cool slightly.

9. Combine the chocolate chips with one tablespoon of coconut oil and melt either over a water bath or in the microwave.

10. Add the warm chickpeas to the melted chocolate and stir well.

11. Line a baking pan with parchment and pour the chocolate mixture into it. Use a spatula to spread the chocolate mixture evenly.

12. Place the baking pan in the refrigerator for a couple of hours to solidify.

13. Once solidified, you can either break or cut the chocolate bark into pieces. Store the pieces in an airtight container until ready to serve.

Pastry Cream with Fruits

This scrumptious pastry cream is sugar-free, making it a perfect PCOS diet dessert. Pair it with the berries of your choice and you have a healthy sweet treat to enjoy after a light (or heavy) meal. Different kinds of berries such as blackberries, strawberries, currants, cranberries, blueberries, and raspberries are full of cancer-fighting, immune-boosting, obesity-preventing, and heart-protecting antioxidants that are beneficial to those suffering from PCOS and other conditions. You can have this pastry cream on its own, with fresh fruits, or add it to other desserts as a topping. It's that versatile!

Nutritional Information for 1 serving:

- Fat: 152.37 g

- Sodium: 0.17 g

- Potassium: 0.35 g

- Protein: 18.22 g

- Fiber: 0.5 g

- Carbs: 27.09 g

- Sugar: 1.31 g

Time: 15 minutes

Serving Size: 1 serving

Ingredients:

- 1 tsp. vanilla extract
- 2 tbsp. arrowhead powder
- ⅓ cup sweetener (powdered)
- ½ cup heavy cream
- 4 eggs (yolks only)
- Berries of choice
- Salt

Directions:

1. In a bowl, combine the arrowhead powder, sweetener, egg yolks, and a pinch of salt. Mix well until you achieve a creamy paste with a light yellow color.

2. In a pot, warm the heavy cream over medium heat until it starts bubbling. When this happens, take the pot off the heat.

3. Add one cup of the hot cream to the egg yolk mixture and mix well to combine.

4. Pour the mixture into the pot, along with the leftover cream. Add the vanilla extract and mix well to combine.

5. Place the pot back on medium heat while whisking constantly. In the beginning, you will have a frothy and thin mixture. Keep whisking until it starts thickening.

6. Once it reaches the consistency of pudding, take the pot off the heat.

7. Gently pour the pastry cream into a strainer for an extra-smooth cream.

8. Pour the strained mixture into a bowl, cover with plastic food wrap, and allow to cool to room temperature.

9. Once cool, place in the refrigerator until ready to serve. To serve, spoon the pastry cream into a bowl and add the fresh berries of your choice.

Smooth Chocolate Ice Cream

Who says you can't enjoy ice cream when you suffer from PCOS? As long as you know how to make your own healthy ice cream, you can enjoy this cold and sweet treat for dessert anytime you want. For this basic recipe, you will be incorporating cashews for extra nutrition, texture, and flavor. Adding nuts to desserts is ideal because nuts are great for improving PCOS symptoms.

According to new research, there are specific components in nuts that improve cholesterol, androgen, and insulin levels in women who suffer from PCOS. This is another simple recipe that teaches you the basic steps for making homemade ice cream. Later, you can substitute some of the ingredients to create different flavors.

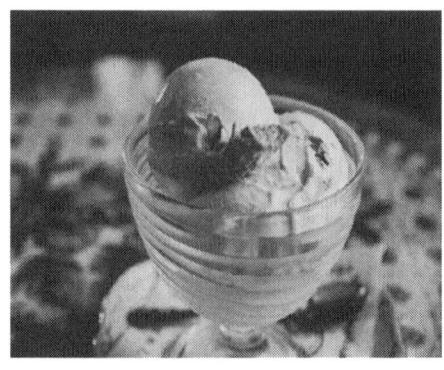

Nutritional Information for 1 scoop of ice cream:

- Fat: 14 g

- Protein: 2 g

- Carbs: 4 g

- Sugar: 2 g

Time: 20 minutes

Serving Size: 1 batch

Ingredients:

- 1 tsp. vanilla extract

- ⅓ cup cacao powder

- ½ cup cashews (raw, soaked for at least 2 hours)

- ¾ cup coconut milk (full-fat)

- ¾ cup sweetener (granulated)

- Sea salt

Directions:

1. In a blender, add the coconut milk and cashews, then blend until you achieve a creamy consistency.

2. Add the rest of the measured ingredients, plus a pinch of sea salt, and continue blending until everything is well combined.

3. Pour the mixture into a Ziplock bag, remove the air, and seal it.

4. Place the Ziplock bag in your freezer for at least 4 hours.

5. Take the Ziplock bag out of the freezer and break up chunks of the frozen ice cream.

6. Place into a food processor and pulse until you achieve a creamy consistency, like soft-serve ice cream.

7. Transfer the soft ice cream into a dish and place back into the freezer for 1 to 3 hours until firm.

8. Once firm, scoop the ice cream into a bowl and serve.

Chapter 8: PCOS Diet Smoothie and Snack Recipes

While following the PCOS diet, you can enjoy occasional snacks whenever you feel hungry. There are so many different kinds of snacks you can enjoy, but make sure to include the calorie content in your daily total. That way, you don't exceed the recommended number of calories per day. The best thing to do if you choose to have a snack in the morning or in the afternoon is to have a light dinner that will complete your caloric intake for the day.

In this chapter, we will focus on smoothies—which you can have for breakfast or as a snack—and other healthy snacks you can prepare in your kitchen. As with the other recipes we have gone through, these all contain healthy ingredients that are beneficial for your condition.

Berry Smoothie

The great thing about this smoothie recipe is that the sweetness comes from the berry content. Berries have a naturally sweet taste but are low in fructose—the unhealthy kind of sugar. This makes them perfect for the PCOS diet. Most berries are rich in antioxidants. In particular, blueberries help increase your insulin sensitivity. These berries are tasty, nutritious, and highly versatile. You can eat them fresh, add them to pastry desserts, and include them in smoothies, too. This is a refreshing smoothie that will fill you up and satisfy your sweet cravings.

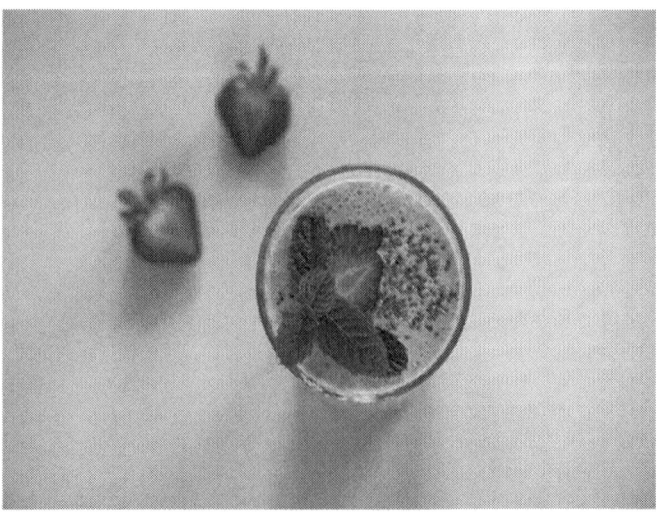

Nutritional Information for 1 smoothie:

- Fat: 21 g

- Protein: 2.5 g

- Fiber: 7.4 g

- Carbs: 19.7 g

- Sugar: 9.8 g

Time: 5 minutes

Serving Size: 1 smoothie

Ingredients:

- ½ cup blueberries (frozen)

- ½ cup coconut cream (full-fat)

- ½ cup raspberries (frozen)

- 1 cup almond milk (unsweetened)

- 1 tbsp. sweetener (optional)

- 1-2 ice cubes (optional)

Directions:

1. In a blender, combine all of the ingredients. Add the sweetener and ice cubes as well, if desired.

2. Blend the ingredients on high for about 1 minute until you achieve a smooth consistency.

3. Serve immediately.

Green Smoothie

This healthy smoothie is chock-full of superfoods. It's a perfect breakfast option and it's an excellent snack, too, if you're craving something healthy and tasty. It's low-carb, high-fat, and even contains potassium and magnesium. Enjoying this smoothie regularly may help you combat various illnesses and diseases. One healthy ingredient in this super smoothie is MCT oil. This type of oil is commonly included in salad dressings, smoothies, and more. It's a healthy oil that increases energy, promotes weight loss, combats yeast and bacterial growth, reduces the risk of heart disease, and helps control blood sugar levels.

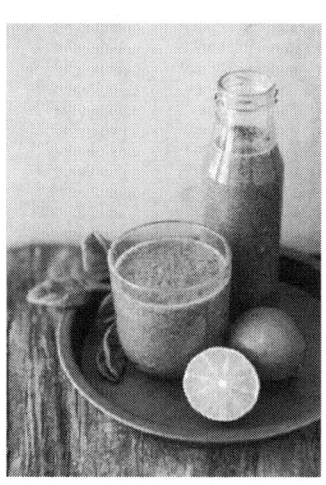

Nutritional Information for 1 smoothie:

- Fat: 36 g

- Sodium: 0.04 g

- Potassium: 0.7 g

- Protein: 5.4 g

- Fiber: 5.4 g

- Carbs: 11.4 g

- Sugar: 1.8 g

Time: 5 minutes

Serving Size: 1 smoothie

Ingredients:

- ½ tsp. vanilla extract (unsweetened)

- 1 tbsp. MCT oil

- 2 tbsp. sweetener (liquid)

- ½ cup coconut milk

- ½ cup spinach (fresh)

- ⅔ cup water

- ½ medium avocado (pitted)

- 1 tsp. matcha powder (optional)

- ¼ cup whey or egg white protein powder (optional)

- 1-2 ice cubes (optional)

Directions:

1. In a blender, add all of the ingredients. Include the matcha powder, protein powder, and ice cubes as well, if desired.

2. Blend the ingredients on high for about 1 minute until you achieve a smooth consistency.

3. Serve immediately.

Piña Colada Smoothie

This protein smoothie is healthy, delicious, easy to make, and packed with protein. It's a refreshing beverage with a tropical flavor, thanks to the pineapple—its main ingredient. Pineapple is great for PCOS because it's rich in an enzyme known as bromelain. When you ingest this enzyme in the proper amounts, it provides some incredible effects. It can help relieve pain, acts as an anticoagulant and blood thinner, and it has anti-inflammatory properties. Pineapples also contain manganese, which helps fight against irritability caused by PCOS and PMS.

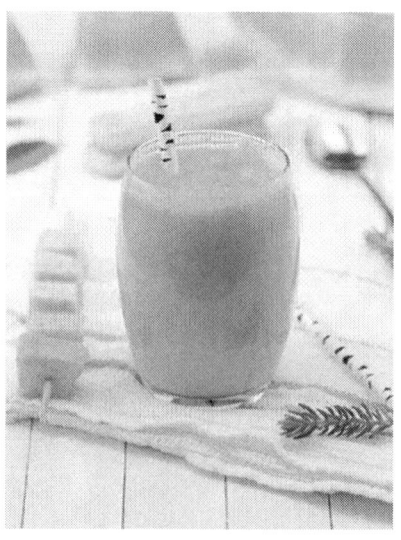

Nutritional Information for 1 smoothie:

- Fat: 8 g
- Sodium: 0.36 g
- Protein: 21 g
- Fiber: 9 g
- Carbs: 32 g
- Sugar: 21 g

Time: 5 minutes

Serving Size: 1 smoothie

Ingredients:

- 1 tsp. honey (raw)
- 1 tsp. vanilla extract
- ½ cup almond milk (vanilla, unsweetened)
- ½ cup coconut milk (unsweetened)
- ¾ cup pineapple chunks (frozen)
- 1 scoop protein powder (vanilla)

Directions:

1. In a blender, add all of the ingredients.

2. Blend the ingredients on high for about 1 minute until you achieve a smooth consistency.

3. Serve immediately.

Mini Quiches

You can eat this winning dish as a light meal or a healthy, hearty snack. It's versatile, easy-to-make, and amazingly savory. Eat this quiche on its own, as a side dish, as an appetizer, or pair it with fresh fruits. One healthy ingredient included in this dish is kale. While raw kale is healthy, if you have PCOS, it's recommended to cook the veggie first. This is because raw kale contains goitrogens that might aggravate your condition. Since you will be cooking the quiche before eating it, you don't have to worry about the kale component. Instead, you can focus on all the healthy nutrients kale (and the other ingredients in this dish) contain.

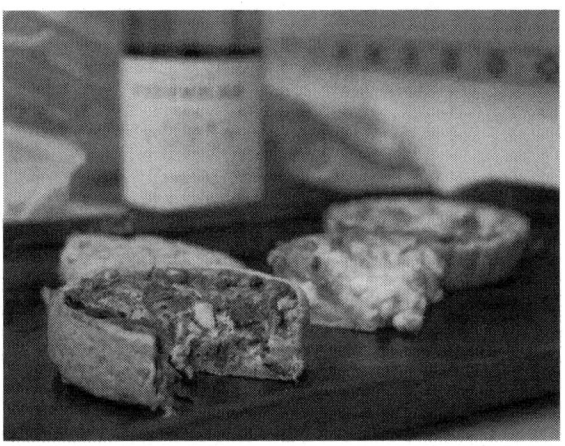

Nutritional Information for 1 quiche:

- Fat: 3 g

- Sodium: 0.11 g

- Protein: 2 g

- Fiber: 1 g

- Carbs: 5 g

Time: 30 minutes

Serving Size: 12 mini quiches

Ingredients:

- ½ tsp. kosher salt

- ¾ tsp. black pepper (freshly ground)

- 2 tbsp. olive oil

- ½ cup quinoa (cooked)

- 1 cup mushrooms (sliced thinly)

- 1 cup water

- ½ medium-sized onion (diced)

- 1 bunch of kale (stems removed, chopped into strips)

- 2 garlic cloves (minced)

- 4 large eggs (beaten)

- Cooking spray

Directions:

1. Preheat your oven to 400°F and grease a muffin pan using cooking spray.

2. In a pan, warm the olive oil over medium heat. Add the onions and mushrooms, then cook for about 10 minutes until caramelized. Stir occasionally to prevent sticking.

3. After cooking, transfer the onions and mushrooms to a bowl.

4. In the same pan, add the kale and cook for about 2 minutes until wilted.

5. Take the kale off the heat and allow to cool. Use a paper towel to remove any excess liquid from the kale.

6. In the bowl with the onions and mushrooms, add the garlic, quinoa, and kale, then stir well to combine. Add the eggs, pepper, and salt, then

continue mixing until well-incorporated.

7. Spoon the mixture into the prepared muffin pan.

8. Place the muffin pan in the oven and bake the mini quiches for about 15 minutes.

9. Take the muffin pan out of the oven and allow the mini quiches to cool for 3 to 5 minutes before serving.

Chocolate Tarts

This decadent chocolate tart is dairy-free, sugar-free, and low-carb. When it comes to creating pastries and baked goods, you may need to perform a lot of substitutions. This is because traditional flours and other types of common baking ingredients have high carb contents. But in this recipe, you will be making use of almond flour—which is nut-based and low-carb. It also adds a nice flavor to the tarts and other baked goods. If you want to stick with your new diet to help improve PCOS symptoms, learning these substitutions is key.

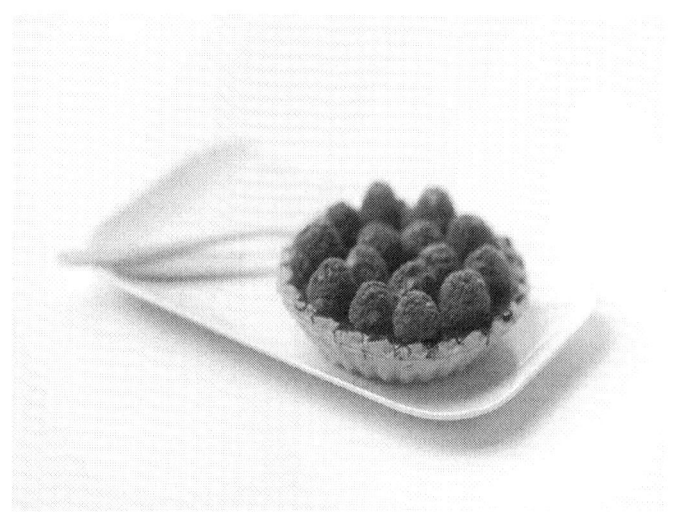

Nutritional Information for 1 slice:

- Fat: 27.34 g

- Sodium: 0.04 g

- Potassium: 0.1 g

- Protein: 9.83 g

- Fiber: 9.8 g

- Carbs: 17.18 g

- Sugar: 3.93 g

Time: 2 hours and 40 minutes

Serving Size: 1 pie tart

Ingredients for the crust:

- 4 tbsp. butter

- ¼ cup sweetener (powdered)

- ½ cup coconut flour

- 1 ½ cups almond flour (blanched)

Ingredients for the mousse and topping:

- 2 tbsp. cocoa powder

- 6 tbsp. sweetener (powdered)

- ¾ cup baking chocolate (unsweetened)

- 1 ⅓ cups coconut milk

- 3 eggs

Directions:

1. Preheat your oven to 350°F and grease a pie tin.

2. In a food processor, combine all of the crust ingredients and pulse until well-combined.

3. Transfer the dough to the pie tin and flatten evenly.

4. Use a fork to stab holes all over the crust—this creates air pockets for when you bake the crust.

5. Place the pie tin in the oven and bake the crust for about 15 minutes.

6. Take the pie tin out of the oven and allow to cool down completely.

7. In a pot, add the coconut milk and bring to a boil. Once it starts boiling, take the pot off the heat and set aside.

8. In a blender, combine the cocoa powder, sweetener, and baking chocolate, then pulse on high to break apart the chocolate.

9. Add the eggs and continue blending until you achieve a thick and creamy consistency.

10. While blending the mixture, take off the lid's small opening and pour the hot coconut milk in slowly and steadily. After you've added all the milk, continue blending for 30 more seconds. This cooks the eggs so you aren't eating them raw.

11. Line the cooled crust with raspberries.

12. Top with the chocolate mousse until you have covered the raspberries completely.

13. Place the chocolate tart in the refrigerator for about 2 hours before slicing and serving. You may also top with more raspberries before serving.

Apple Fritters

If you're craving for something sweet and crispy, this is the recipe for you. As with the other recipes, this one is healthy, easy, and scrumptious, too. For this recipe, apples are the star. Apples are great because they are high in fiber and low in calories. They contain vitamin A, vitamin B6, vitamin C, phosphorus, calcium, iron, potassium, and magnesium. When you eat a lot of fiber, this gives your levels of sex hormone-binding globulin a boost. This, in turn, helps your body fight against testosterone and other types of free hormones that may aggravate PCOS.

Nutritional Information for 1 fritter:

- Fat: 25.7 g

- Sodium: 0.13 g

- Potassium: 0.16 g

- Protein: 3.4 g

- Fiber: 3.2 g

- Carbs: 17.1 g

- Sugar: 11.3 g

Time: 45 minutes

Serving Size: 7 fritters (depending on the size)

Ingredients:

- ½ tsp. baking soda
- ¾ tsp. cinnamon
- 1 tsp. lemon juice
- 1 tsp. vanilla extract
- 1 tbsp. chia seeds (white)
- 2 tbsp. coconut flour
- 3 tbsp. coconut butter
- 5 tbsp. sweetener (liquid)
- ¼ cup coconut milk
- ¼ cup coconut oil
- ½ cup almond flour
- 1 cup apples (diced)
- 1 medium egg
- Sea salt

Directions:

1. Preheat your oven to 350°F and line a baking sheet with parchment paper.

2. In a skillet, add some coconut oil, the chopped apple, cinnamon, and vanilla extract, then sauté on medium heat. Cook for about 7 minutes while stirring frequently.

3. Take the skillet off the heat and set aside.

4. In a bowl, combine the chia seeds, sweetener, baking soda, coconut flour, almond flour, coconut milk, and a pinch of salt, then mix well.

5. Add the cooked apples and continue mixing to combine well.

6. In a sauté pan, warm 2 tablespoons of coconut oil over medium heat.

7. Once the oil has heated up, spoon the apple mixture into the pan. Continue adding spoonfuls of the mixture, making sure to flatten each fritter with the back of your

spoon. Cook the fritters for about 2 minutes on each side.

8. After cooking, transfer the fritters on the baking sheet you have prepared. You may garnish the top with a few pieces of apple.

9. Place the baking sheet in the oven and bake the fritters for 10 to 15 minutes.

10. While the fritters are baking, prepare the sauce.

11. In a pan, combine 3 tablespoons each of coconut oil and coconut butter. Add 2 tablespoons of sweetener and mix until it thickens.

12. Take the baking sheet out of the oven and drizzle the fritters with the sauce. Serve while warm.

Conclusion: Overcoming PCOS Through Your Diet

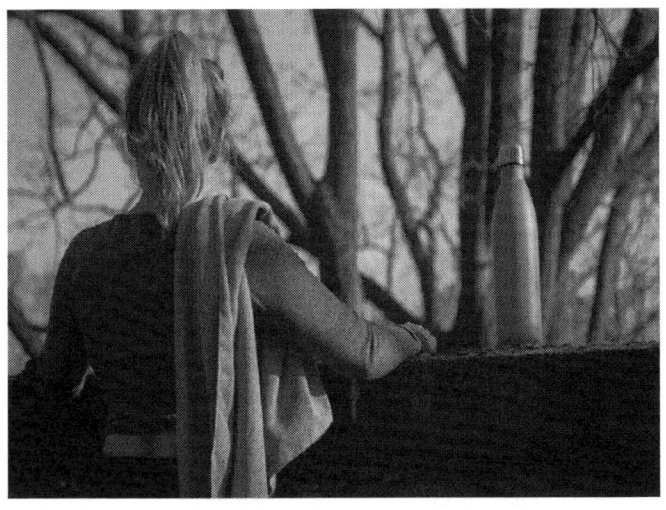

There you have it—all of the basic information you need to know about PCOS and using the PCOS diet to manage your condition more effectively. We started off by defining the condition, including its risk factors, causes, and symptoms. This information helps you become more aware of what you need to look out for so you can determine when it is time to see a doctor—whether for yourself or for someone in your family.

While PCOS is an incurable condition, you can manage, improve, or even put it into remission by following a healthier lifestyle and eating a better diet—specifically, the PCOS diet. We've gone through a wealth of information in this book, and with all you have learned, you may want to leave a positive review for other women who are looking for an informative, interesting, and enlightening book about the PCOS diet.

After learning about the condition, we moved on to the PCOS diet—what it is, the pros and cons, the benefits of following the diet, and what makes this diet stand out from the rest. Since PCOS is associated with other conditions, we discussed those, as well. In particular, we learned how the PCOS diet can be helpful for controlling diabetes, weight loss, and infertility. Then we moved on to practical tips, pointers, and strategies for starting and following the PCOS diet. We even went through a shopping list of ingredients and food items to give you a better idea of what to look for when you're following this diet. Then we finished off the informative section by discussing the basics of meal planning.

All the chapters that followed included a number of healthy, yummy, and simple recipes that you can start whipping up in your kitchen right now. We included breakfast, lunch, dinner, dessert, and snack recipes—all of which contained PCOS diet-friendly ingredients which also happen to be readily available in supermarkets and health stores.

Now that you have reached the end of the book, you are armed with practical information that can help you combat your condition. It's time to take back control over your life by embarking on your PCOS diet journey now! Good luck!

24905130R00090